ADA POCKET GUIDE TO

Lipid Disorders, Hypertension, Diabetes, and Weight Management

UPDATED EDITION (2012)

Marion J. Franz, MS, RD, CDE

Jackie L. Boucher, MS, RD, CDE

Raquel Franzini Pereira, MS, RD

eat right. Academy of Nutrition and Dietetics

Diana Faulhaber, Publisher
Laura Pelehach, Acquisitions and Development Manager
Elizabeth Nishiura, Production Manager

10 9 8 7 6 5 4 3 2 1
ISBN 978-0-88091-461-1

Library of Congress Cataloging-in-Publication Data for 2011 edition

Franz, Marion J.
    ADA pocket guide to lipid disorders, hypertension, diabetes, and
weight management / Marion J. Franz, Jackie L. Boucher, Raquel
Franzini Pereira.
        p. ; cm.
    Other title: Pocket guide to lipid disorders, hypertension, diabetes,
and weight management
    Includes bibliographical references and index.
    ISBN 978-0-88091-447-5
    1. Diet therapy—Handbooks, manuals, etc. 2. Lipids—Metabolism—
Disorders—Diet therapy—Handbooks, manuals, etc. 3. Hypertension—
Diet therapy—Handbooks, manuals, etc. 4. Diabetes—Diet therapy
—Handbooks, manuals, etc. 5. Reducing diets—Handbooks, manuals,
etc. I. Boucher, Jackie. II. Pereira, Raquel Franzini. III. American
Dietetic Association. IV. Title. V. Title: Pocket guide to lipid disorders,
hypertension, diabetes, and weight management.
    [DNLM: 1. Lipid Metabolism Disorders—diet therapy—Handbooks.
2. Diabetes Mellitus—diet therapy—Handbooks. 3. Hypertension—
diet therapy—Handbooks. 4. Nutrition Assessment—Handbooks.
5. Nutrition Therapy—Handbooks. 6. Obesity—diet therapy—
Handbooks. WD 200.1]
    RM216.F83 2011
    615.8'54—dc22
                                                        2010027170

Contents

Tables

Reviewers

Theresa M. Dildy, MS, RD
St. Luke's Episcopal Health Hospital
Houston, TX

Michele M. Doucette, PhD
University of Colorado School of Medicine
Golden, CO

Alison Evert, MS, RD, CDE
University of Washington Medical Center—Diabetes
   Care Center
Woodinville, WA

Molly Gee, MEd, RD
Baylor College of Medicine
Houston, TX

Kirsten F. Hilpert, PhD, RD
State University of New York—College of Oneonta
Oneonta, NY

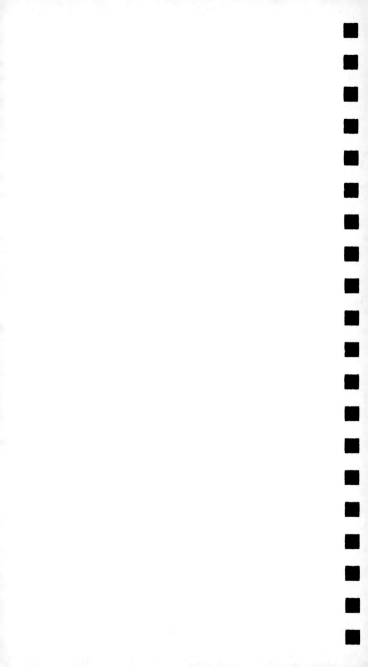

Frequently Used Abbreviations

A1C	hemoglobin A1c
ACEI	angiotensin converting enzyme inhibitor
ADI	acceptable daily intake
ARB	angiotensin receptor blocker
BB	beta blocker
BG	blood glucose
BMI	body mass index
BP	blood pressure
CAD	coronary artery disease
CCB	calcium channel blockers
CGM	continuous glucose monitoring
CHD	coronary heart disease
CHF	congestive heart failure
CKD	chronic kidney disease
CRP	C-reactive protein
CVD	cardiovascular disease
DASH	Dietary Approaches to Stop Hypertension
DB	diabetes
DBP	diastolic blood pressure
DHA	docosahexaenoic acid
DRI	Dietary Reference Intake
DSMT	diabetes self management training
EAL	Evidence Analysis Library
EBNPG	Evidence-Based Nutrition Practice Guidelines
EPA	eicosapentaenoic acid
FDA	Food and Drug Administration
FPG	fasting plasma glucose

GDM	gestational diabetes mellitus
GFR	glomerular filtration rate
GI	gastrointestinal
HDL-C	high-density lipoprotein cholesterol
HTN	hypertension
IDNT	International Dietetics and Nutrition Terminology
IFG	impaired fasting glucose
IGT	impaired glucose tolerance
JNC 7	Joint National Committee on Prevention, Detection, Evaluation and Treatment of High Blood Pressure
LD	lipid disorders
LDL-C	low-density lipoprotein cholesterol
MET	metabolic equivalent
MI	myocardial infarction
MNT	medical nutrition therapy
NCEP-ATP III	National Cholesterol Education Program-Adult Treatment Panel III
NCP	Nutrition Care Process
NHLBI	National Heart, Lung, and Blood Institute
OGTT	oral glucose tolerance test
OTC	over the counter
PES	problem, etiology, signs and symptoms
PG	plasma glucose
PPG	peak postprandial glucose
RD	registered dietitian
RMR	resting metabolic rate
SBP	systolic blood pressure
SFA	saturated fatty acids
SMBG	self-monitoring of blood glucose
TC	total cholesterol

TEE	total energy expenditure
TG	triglycerides
TLC	therapeutic lifestyle change
VLDL	very low–density lipoprotein
WC	waist circumference
WM	weight management

Criteria for the Rating of Evidence-Based Nutrition Recommendations

Strong: The benefits of the recommendation approach clearly exceed the harms (or the harms clearly exceed the benefits in the case of a negative recommendation) and the quality of the supporting evidence is excellent/good (grade I or II).

Fair: The benefits of the recommendation approach clearly exceed the harms (or the harms clearly exceed the benefits in the case of a negative recommendation) but the quality of the evidence is not as strong (grade II or III).

Weak: The quality of the evidence that exists is either suspect or in well-done studies (grade I, II, or III) shows little clear advantage to one approach vs another.

Consensus: The expert opinion (grade IV) supports the guideline recommendation even though the available scientific evidence did not present consistent results, or controlled trials were lacking.

Insufficient evidence: Lack of pertinent evidence (grade V) and/or an unclear balance between benefits and harms.

Source: Data are from reference 1.

Preface

Lipid disorders, hypertension, diabetes, overweight, and obesity are common medical problems. Registered dietitians (RDs) and other health professionals see patients with these conditions, or combinations of these conditions, daily. To assist RDs in providing high-quality, evidence-based nutrition care, this pocket guide addresses nutrition care for each of these conditions. The purpose of this pocket guide is to integrate information from various Academy of Nutrition and Dietetics (formerly American Dietetic Association/ADA) resources, including evidence-based nutrition practice guidelines (EBNPG) (1), toolkits, the *International Dietetics & Nutrition Terminology (IDNT) Reference Manual: Standardized Language for the Nutrition Care Process* (2), and scope and standards of practice (3). The pocket guide does not replace these in-depth resources. Instead, it abbreviates the information and aims to help RDs provide nutrition care for individuals with lipid disorders, hypertension, diabetes, and/or overweight or obesity. Because it is common to educate and counsel clients/patients with more than one of these conditions, the pocket guide provides suggestions as to how to provide nutrition care for individuals with multiple medical problems. RDs who work in clinic, inpatient, and public health settings will find the content of the guide to be useful in their clinical practice.

The publication of this guide would not be possible without the efforts and accomplishments of many others. The Academy of Nutrition and Dietetics has provided vision and support for the development of EBNPG, the Nutrition Care Process (NCP), and standardized language.

Without this support, none of these projects could have been accomplished. Special mention must be given to Esther Myers, PhD, RD, FADA, and Academy staff for their guidance and persistence in the development of standardized language and the Nutrition Care Process. The dietetics profession is indebted to all of the many members who contributed, and continue to contribute, to the NCP and IDNT, which together provide the framework for nutrition care. Guidance and support for EBNPG is provided by the Academy of Nutrition and Dietetics Evidence-Based Practice Committee. They oversee the evidence analysis process, maintenance of the Evidence Analysis Library, and the development of all EBNPG and toolkits. We thank the many Academy members who have contributed their expertise and time to these projects. In particular, we acknowledge Deborah Cummins, PhD, Kari Kren, MPH, RD, other staff members, and the Academy member analysts without whom none of these projects would have reached completion.

We also express our sincere appreciation to Laura Pelehach, acquisitions and development manager for the Academy's book publishing team. Without her vision, expertise, and support, this guide would not have been written. A very special word of appreciation and thanks to the reviewers and editors for their suggestions and comments; we have incorporated them into the guide. To all who participated in the process and development of this guide, we express our sincere thanks and gratitude!

MARION J. FRANZ, MS, RD, CDE
JACKIE L. BOUCHER, MS, RD, CDE
RAQUEL FRANZINI PEREIRA, MS, RD

Chapter 1

Evidence-Based Nutrition Practice and the Nutrition Care Process

HOW TO NAVIGATE THIS POCKET GUIDE

This pocket guide is organized to follow the steps in the Nutrition Care Process (NCP)—nutrition assessment, nutrition diagnosis, nutrition intervention, and nutrition monitoring and evaluation (2,4). Integrated with the NCP are the Academy of Nutrition and Dietetics (formerly American Dietetic Association/ADA) evidence-based nutrition practice guidelines (EBNPG) for lipid disorders (5), hypertension (6), type 1 and type 2 diabetes (7,8), gestational diabetes (9), and weight management (10), which are published in the Academy of Nutrition and Dietetics Evidence Analysis Library (1) and the *Journal of the Academy of Nutrition and Dietetics*. Registered dietitians (RDs) can use this guide to find concise and essential information needed to plan, implement, monitor/evaluate, and document nutrition care provided in clinic, inpatient, and public health settings. In subsequent chapters, the relevant EBNPG are noted in the parentheses using this key:

- **LD** = lipid disorders
- **HTN** = hypertension
- **DB** = diabetes
- **WM** = weight management

This guide draws primarily from two sources: the EBNPG and the Academy's *International Dietetics & Nutrition Terminology (IDNT) Reference Manual* for standardized language (2). The evidence analysis process used to develop the EBNPG is a rigorous and systematic process for searching, analyzing, and summarizing research on a specific nutrition topic. From the evidence summaries and conclusion statements, evidence-based nutrition recommendations and guidelines are developed. In this pocket guide, recommendations from the EBNPG are organized by the section of the NCP to which they apply—nutrition assessment (Chapter 2), nutrition diagnosis (Chapter 3), nutrition intervention (Chapters 4 and 5), and nutrition monitoring and evaluation (Chapter 6).

This guide also aids in the essential integration of medical nutrition therapy (MNT) into the overall medical management of health problems. In addition to EBNPG conclusions, subsequent chapters include recommendations from the National Cholesterol Education Program (11); American Heart Association (12,13); Joint National Committee on Prevention, Detection, and Evaluation and Treatment of High Blood Pressure (14); American Diabetes Association (15); American Association of Clinical Endocrinologists (16); National Heart, Lung, and Blood Institute (17); US Department of Health and Human Services (18); and American College of Sports Medicine (19).

Chapter 2 integrates the EBNPG into the first step in the NCP, nutrition assessment (and reassessment for follow-up nutrition care), in which the RD obtains and collects timely and appropriate data, and analyzes and interprets the data with evidence-based standards. Chapter 3 reviews the second NCP step, nutrition diagnosis, which involves identifying and labeling nutrition-related problems, determining the problems' cause and contributing

risk factors, clustering signs and symptoms, and defin-
ing the problems' characteristics. Examples of possible
nutrition diagnoses and PES (problem, etiology, signs and
symptoms) statements for conditions are given.

Chapters 4 and 5 cover step 3 in the NCP, nutrition
intervention, which involves planning (formulating goals
and determining plans of action) so that nutrition interventions are integrated into overall disease management
and implementation (care delivered and action carried
out). Chapter 4 summarizes the development of nutrition
prescriptions for MNT as part of disease management.
Chapter 5 summarizes EBNPG recommendations related
to nutrition education and outlines nutrition counseling
strategies used to implement the nutrition prescription and
recommendations.

Chapter 6 summarizes the critical fourth NCP step,
nutrition monitoring and evaluation, which involves
monitoring progress, measuring outcome indicators,
and evaluating outcomes. This requires that RDs know
expected outcomes of nutrition interventions for the treatment and prevention of chronic diseases. Documentation
is also reviewed in Chapter 6.

EXPECTED OUTCOMES FROM
MEDICAL NUTRITION THERAPY

Lipid Disorders

Elevated LDL cholesterol (LDL-C), total cholesterol
(TC), triglyceride (TG), and low HDL cholesterol (HDL-
C) concentrations are risk factors for cardiovascular diseases (CVD) including coronary heart disease (CHD),
coronary artery disease (CAD), hypertension and stroke.
Scientific evidence strongly supports the effectiveness
of MNT as a means to manage dyslipidemia and reduce

risk factors associated with CVD. Cardioprotective nutrition therapy can reduce TC by 7% to 21%, LDL-C by 7% to 22%, and triglycerides by 11% to 31% (5). Patients who attend multiple RD visits for MNT can reduce daily dietary fat intake by 5% to 8%, saturated fat intake by 2% to 4%, and energy intake by 235 to 700 kcal/day, which contributes to the positive outcomes cited (5,20). The combined intervention of a cardioprotective eating pattern, increased physical activity, and a 7% to 10% weight loss is also effective for preventing and treating metabolic syndrome, which is a clustering of risk factors for CVD that includes dyslipidemia (12).

Hypertension

Hypertension in adults is a major risk factor for CVD and stroke. Lifestyle modifications reduce blood pressure (BP) in both normotensive and hypertensive adults, improve the effectiveness of antihypertensive drugs, and reduce CVD risk (21). Some lifestyle modifications can reduce BP as well as single-drug therapy. Implementation of multiple lifestyle interventions can lead to substantial, clinically relevant reductions in blood pressure (13). When hypertensive individuals not on medication followed major lifestyle recommendations—weight loss, sodium reduction, increased physical activity, and the Dietary Approaches to Stop Hypertension (DASH) diet, which is rich in fruits, vegetables, and low-fat dairy products but low in saturated and total fat—their systolic blood pressure (SBP) was reduced by 14.2 mmHg and diastolic blood pressure (DBP) by 7.4 mmHg. The same intervention in nonhypertensive individuals decreased SBP and DBP by 9.2 mmHg and 5.8 mmHg, respectively (22). In general, studies implementing MNT provided by RDs for hypertension report an average reduction in blood pressure of approximately 5 mmHg for both SBP and DBP (23).

Diabetes

Type 1 diabetes is primarily a disease of insulin deficiency whereas type 2 diabetes is a progressive disease that results from defects in insulin action (insulin resistance) and insulin secretion (insulin deficiency). Diabetes is diagnosed when an individual's endogenous insulin is insufficient to overcome the insulin resistance and he or she develops hyperglycemia. Diabetes MNT provided by RDs can effectively decrease hemoglobin A1c (A1C) by approximately 1% to 2% (range = –0.5% to –2.6%), depending on the type, duration of diabetes, and level of glycemic control (7,24). MNT has the greatest impact following the initial diagnosis and continues to be effective throughout the disease process. Outcomes of nutrition interventions are generally measurable in 6 weeks to 3 months, and evaluation by an A1C test should be done at this time. If a patient's glycemic control has not clinically improved at 3 months, the RD should contact the referral source and recommend the need for a change in medication(s).

Lifestyle interventions can prevent or delay the development of type 2 diabetes in persons with pre-diabetes (25). In the first 2.8 years of the Diabetes Prevention Program (DPP), diabetes incidence in high-risk adults was reduced 58% by intensive lifestyle intervention (a reduced-energy diet, physical activity, and weight-reduction targets) and 31% by metformin only compared with placebo (26). In the 10-year follow-up to DPP, participants in the original lifestyle-intervention arm had maintained their low rate of diabetes onset (27). Similar results were reported in the 7-year follow-up of subjects in the Finnish Diabetes Prevention Study (28).

Overweight and Obesity

Overweight and obesity are complex, multifactorial chronic diseases that develop from an interaction between genetics and the environment and are associated with increased morbidity and mortality (29). An overweight or obese individual's health can improve with relatively modest weight losses of 5% to 10% of body weight. A mean weight loss of 5 to 8.5 kg (5% to 9%) can be expected during the first 6 months from interventions involving a reduced-energy diet and/or weight-loss medications, with weight plateaus at approximately 6 months (30). Although maintenance of weight loss is a greater challenge than weight loss, a mean weight loss of 3 to 6 kg (3% to 6%) can be maintained when individuals receive continued support (30,31).

PLANNING NUTRITION ENCOUNTERS

Multiple encounters between the RD and a client/patient are required to implement nutrition interventions that will facilitate the goals of nutrition therapy and achieve desirable outcomes. The EBNPG for lipid disorders, hypertension, diabetes, and weight management provide encounter guidelines, which are described in the sections that follow. The rating of each recommendation is listed parenthetically after the recommendation (see page xv for rating definitions). Note that for clients/patients who present with multiple health issues, the RD must decide whether nutrition care can be provided by following the guidelines for the primary disease process or if additional encounters will be needed.

Lipid Disorders (5)

• Multiple RD visits for MNT lasting an average of 45 minutes (30 to 60 minutes per session) over 6 to 12 weeks are recommended for individuals with an abnormal lipid profile (see Table 2.1 in Chapter 2) or for individuals with CHD. (Strong)

- More than 2 visits for MNT (3 to 6 visits) are recommended. (Fair)
- If a patient is taking lipid-lowering medications, three or more visits for MNT averaging 45 minutes per session over a 6- to 8-week period are recommended. (Fair)

Hypertension (6)

- A comprehensive program including lifestyle modification (weight reduction, MNT, and physical activity) and pharmacologic therapy is recommended for the management of elevated BP. (Consensus)

Diabetes (7,8)

- An initial series of three or four encounters (45–90 minutes each) with an RD for MNT is recommended. This series, beginning at the diagnosis of diabetes or at first referral to an RD for MNT for diabetes, should be completed within 3 to 6 months. The RD should determine whether additional MNT encounters are needed after the initial series. (Strong)
- At least one follow-up encounter is recommended annually to reinforce lifestyle changes and evaluate and monitor outcomes that indicate the need for changes in MNT or medication. The RD should determine whether additional MNT encounters are needed. (Strong)
- The RD should implement and coordinate care with an interdisciplinary team. (Consensus)

Weight Management (10)

- Weight loss and weight maintenance therapy based on a comprehensive weight management program that includes diet, physical activity, and behavior therapy is recommended. (Strong)

- MNT for weight loss should last at least 6 months or until weight loss goals are achieved, with implementation of a weight maintenance program after that time. (Strong)

PRIORITIZING AND COMBINING MEDICAL NUTRITION THERAPY

For persons with lipid disorders, initial MNT recommendations are for 25% to 35% of energy intake from total fat, less than 7% of energy intake from saturated fatty acids and *trans* fatty acids, and less than 200 mg of food cholesterol per day (5). If hypertension is a concurrent problem, a sodium intake limited to no more than 2,300 mg per day and a DASH eating pattern are recommended (6).

For people with type 1, type 2, or gestational diabetes, MNT begins with interventions shown to improve glycemic outcomes (7–9). Glucose control improves soon after MNT is implemented, and these improvements encourage individuals to continue lifestyle interventions. A variety of interventions (reduced energy and fat intake, carbohydrate counting, simplified meal plans, healthy food choices, individualized meal-planning strategies, exchange lists, insulin-to-carbohydrate ratios, low-fat vegan diets, physical activity, and behavioral strategies) have been shown to be effective (7). People with diabetes frequently also have lipid disorders and hypertension. MNT interventions for these problems should also be implemented in the initial series of encounters.

Successful weight loss and weight management therapies can help prevent or delay type 2 diabetes (25–28), hypertension (13), metabolic syndrome, and elevated triglycerides (12,32). Therefore, an energy-controlled food pattern and regular physical activity are important components of MNT for these conditions.

CONCLUSION

When clients have only one medical diagnosis, disease-specific recommendations are available in the Academy's Evidence Analysis Library (EAL) (1). A major goal of this pocket guide, however, is to help RDs integrate the EBNPG for lipid disorders, hypertension, diabetes, and adult weight management as well as MNT for pre-diabetes and metabolic syndrome into individualized nutrition care for clients/patients who have multiple medical diagnoses. Along with information from the referral source, laboratory data, the individual's food/nutrition history, and client/patient preferences, the RD can use this pocket guide to prioritize nutrition therapy interventions that will be most effective in reducing risk of disease complications.

Chapter 2

Nutrition Assessment

The Nutrition Care Process begins with nutrition assessment. Assessment data are available from the referral source, the patient's medical records, and the patient/client. Prior to the first encounter, data can be compiled from the patient's medical records, forms the patient completes, and information received from the referral source. It is essential to know the patient's medical condition(s) for which MNT is requested (Tables 2.1–2.8), the goals of therapy (Tables 2.9–2.12, 2.14), and the medications prescribed for the medical conditions(s) (Tables 2.21–2.43). By collecting as much data as possible before the first encounter, implementation of education/counseling can begin more efficiently.

It is also helpful at the beginning of the MNT encounter to determine why the patient/client has scheduled the appointment and his or her questions. A patient's reply to a question such as "What brought you here today?" can help determine his or her readiness to change. For example, the reply "My doctor told me to come" requires different education and counseling strategies than the reply "I asked my doctor for a referral." A second question—"Do you have questions or goals for our session today?"—will help tailor the encounter so that the patient's concerns are addressed. (See the nutrition counseling section in Chapter 5.)

This chapter does not cover *all* assessment data that might be needed, but the various tables highlight important assessment parameters related to lipid disorders, hypertension, diabetes, and weight management. The order in which the assessment data are collected will vary depending on individual circumstances and needs. Furthermore, nutrition assessment is an ongoing process that involves data collection at initial and follow-up encounters and ongoing analysis of patient/client data and needs. The particular EBNPG to which the assessment applies are noted parenthetically, using this key:

- **LD** = lipid disorders
- **HTN** = hypertension
- **DB** = diabetes
- **WM** = weight management

Other abbreviations are listed on page xi.

The following nutrition assessment domains (categories) are important for the implementation of nutrition therapy for lipid disorders, hypertension, diabetes, and weight management (2):

- **Biochemical Data, Medical Tests, and Procedures**, which include laboratory data for lipids, glucose, kidney function, and other nutrition-related tests
- **Nutrition-Focused Physical Findings**, which includes vital signs such as blood pressure
- **Anthropometric Measurements**, which include height, weight, BMI, waist circumference or waist-to-hip ratio, growth rate (in children), and rate of weight change
- **Client History**, which includes the following:
  - General patient/client information, such as age, gender, race/ethnicity, language, literacy, and education
  - Medical/health history and medical treatment, including goals of medical therapy and prescribed medications related to the medical condition for which MNT is being implemented

  ○ Social history, such as social and medical support, cultural and religious beliefs, and socioeconomic status
  ○ Patient/client or family nutrition-related medical/ health history
  ○ Other medical or surgical treatments, and complementary/alternative medicine
- **Food/Nutrition-Related History**, including food and beverage intake; energy and macronutrient intake; meal-snack pattern; bioactive substances (eg, alcohol intake, use of fish oil); nutrition and health knowledge, beliefs, and behaviors; food availability; physical activity; and readiness to change nutrition-related behaviors
- **Energy and Macronutrient Needs**, which are compared with assessment of food and nutrient intake to assist in determining relevant nutrition diagnoses and nutrition interventions

BIOCHEMICAL DATA, MEDICAL TESTS, AND DIAGNOSTIC CRITERIA

Assessment of biochemical data, medical tests, and diagnostic criteria helps to identify medical conditions and nutrition-related medical concerns associated with the following:

- LDL-C, TC, HDL-C, TG (LD, HTN, DB, WM) [Table 2.1]
- Metabolic syndrome (LD, HTN, DB, WM) [Table 2.2]
- Blood pressure (HTN, DB, LD, WM) [Table 2.3]
- Glycemia and A1C (DB) [Table 2.4 and Table 2.5]
- Albumin excretion and stages of chronic kidney disease (DB and, if appropriate, HTN) [Table 2.6 and Table 2.7]

Table 2.1 Classification of LDL, Total, and HDL Cholesterol; Triglycerides; and C-Reactive Protein

LDL-C[a]

- Optimal: <100 mg/dL (2.6 mmol/L)
- Near or above optimal: 100–129 mg/dL (2.6–3.3 mmol/L)
- Borderline high: 130–159 mg/dL (3.4–4.1 mmol/L)
- High: 160–189 mg/dL (4.2–4.9 mmol/L)
- Very high: ≥190 mg/dL (5.0 mmol/L)

TC

- Desirable: <200 mg/dL (5.2 mmol/L)
- Borderline high: 200–239 mg/dL (5.2–6.2 mmol/L)
- High: ≥240 mg/dL (6.2 mmol/L)

HDL-C

- Low: <40 mg/dL (0.9 mmol/L) in men; <50 mg/dL (1.1 mmol/L) in women
- High: ≥60 mg/dL (1.1 mmol/L)

TG[b]

- Normal: <150 mg/dL (1.7 mmol/L)
- Borderline high: 150–199 mg/dL (1.7–2.2 mmol/L)
- High: 200–499 mg/dL (2.3–5.6 mmol/L)
- Very high: ≥500 mg/dL (5.7 mmol/L)

CRP

- Low risk: <1.0 mg/dL
- Average risk: 1.0–3.0 mg/dL
- High risk >3.0 mg/dL

[a]An LDL-C goal of <70 mg/dL (1.8 mmol/L) is a reasonable strategy for persons who have diabetes or overt CVD or are considered to be at extremely high risk for these diseases.
[b]If TG are ≥200 mg/dL (2.3 mmol/L), non-HDL-C should be <130 mg/dL (3.4 mmol/L) (non-HDL-C = TC – HDL-C).
Source: Data are from references 33 and 34.

Table 2.2   Diagnostic Criteria[a] for Metabolic Syndrome

Elevated WC[b]

- Men: >40 inches (102 cm)
- Women: >35 inches (88 cm)

Elevated TG

- ≥ 150 mg/dL (1.7 mmol/L)

    or

- Drug treatment for elevated TG

Reduced HDL-C

- Men: <40 mg/dL (0.9 mmol/L)
- Women: <50 mg/dL (1.1 mmol/L)

    or

- Drug treatment for reduced HDL-C

Elevated BP

- ≥130 mmHg SBP

    or

- ≥85 mmHg DBP

    or

- Drug treatment for hypertension

Elevated FPG

- ≥100 mg/dL (5.6 mmol/L)

    or

- Drug treatment for elevated glucose

---

[a]Any 3 of 5 criteria constitute diagnosis.

[b]A lower cutpoint for elevated WC (eg, ≥35 inches [90 cm] in men and ≥31 inches [80 cm] in women) seems appropriate for Asian Americans; other population- and country-specific definitions are listed in reference 35.

Source: Adapted with permission from reference 35: Alberti KGMM, Eckel RH, Grundy SM, Zimmet PZ, Cleeman JI, Donato KA, Fruchart JC, James PT, Loria CM, Smith Jr, SC. Harmonizing the metabolic syndrome. A Joint Interim Statement of the International Diabetes Federation Task Force on Epidemiology and Prevention; National Heart, Lung and Blood Institute; American Heart Association; World Health Federation; International Atherosclerosis Society; and International Association for the Study of Obesity. *Circulation*. 2009;120:1640–1645.

Table 2.3 Classification of Blood Pressure in Adults

Classification[a]	Blood Pressure, mmHg	Lifestyle Modification
Normal	SBP <120 *and* DBP <80	Encourage
Prehypertension	SBP 120–139 *or* DBP 80–89	Yes
Stage 1 hypertension	SBP 140–159 *or* DBP 90–99	Yes
Stage 2 hypertension	SBP ≥160 *or* DBP ≥100	Yes

[a]Based on mean of data from two or more seated BP readings on each of two or more office visits.

Source: Adapted from reference 36: The Seventh Report of the Joint National Committee on Prevention, Detection, Evaluation and Treatment of High Blood Pressure: The JNC 7 Report. Bethesda, MD: National Institutes of Heart, Lung, and Blood Institute; 2003. NIH publication 03-5231.

Table 2.4 Criteria for the Diagnosis of Diabetes

1. A1C ≥6.5%. Test standardized to the Diabetes Control and Complications Trial assay.[a]
   or
2. FPG ≥126 mg/dL (7.0 mmol/L). Fasting, no caloric intake for at least 8 h.[a]
   or
3. Two-hour plasma glucose ≥200 mg/dL (11.1 mmol/L) during an OGTT. A glucose load containing the equivalent of 75 g anhydrous glucose dissolved in water should be used.[a]
   or
4. Classic symptoms of hyperglycemia or hyperglycemic crisis and a random PG ≥200 mg/dL (11.1 mmol/L).

[a]In the absence of unequivocal hyperglycemia, criteria 1–3 should be confirmed by repeat testing. A1C assay should not be used during pregnancy for diagnosis of diabetes as changes in red cell turnover make the A1C problematic; PG measurements are required.

Source: Adapted with permission from American Diabetes Association. Standards of medical care in diabetes—2010. *Diabetes Care*. 2010;33(suppl 1): S11–S61. These data are also found in the reference 15: American Diabetes Association. Standards of medical care in diabetes—2012. *Diabetes Care*. 2012;35(suppl 1):S11–S63.

Table 2.5 Categories of Increased Risk for Diabetes (Prediabetes)[a]

- FPG: 100–125 mg/dL (5.6–6.9 mmol/L) = IFG
- 2-h PG on the 75-g OGTT: 140–199 mg/dL (7.8–11.0 mmol/L) = IGT
- A1C 5.7%–6.4%

[a]For all three tests, risk is continuous, extending below the lower limit of the range and becoming disproportionately greater at higher ends of the range.

Source: Adapted with permission from American Diabetes Association. Standards of medical care in diabetes—2010. *Diabetes Care.* 2010; 33(suppl 1):S11–S61. These data are also found in the reference 15: American Diabetes Association. Standards of medical care in diabetes—2012. *Diabetes Care.* 2012;35(suppl 1):S11–S63.

Table 2.6 Definitions of Abnormalities in Albumin Excretion

Category	Spot Collection, mcg/mg Creatinine
Normal	<30
Microalbuminuria	30–299
Macroalbuminuria (clinical)	≥300

Source: Reprinted with permission from American Diabetes Association. Standards of medical care in diabetes—2010. *Diabetes Care.* 2010;33 (suppl 1):S11–S61. These data are also found in the reference 15: American Diabetes Association. Standards of medical care in diabetes—2012. *Diabetes Care.* 2012;35(suppl 1):S11–S63.

Table 2.7 Stages of Chronic Kidney Disease

Stage	Description	GFR, mL/min per 1.73 m^2 body surface area
1	Kidney damage[a] with normal or increased GFR	≥90
2	Kidney damage[a] with mildly decreased GFR	60–89
3	Moderately decreased GFR	30–59
4	Severely decreased GFR	15–29
5	Kidney failure	<15 or dialysis

[a]Kidney damage defined as abnormalities on pathologic, urine, blood, or imaging tests.

Source: Reprinted with permission from American Diabetes Association. Standards of medical care in diabetes—2010. *Diabetes Care.* 2010;33 (suppl 1):S11–S61. These data are also found in the reference 15: American Diabetes Association. Standards of medical care in diabetes—2012. *Diabetes Care.* 2012;35(suppl 1):S11–S63.

ANTHROPOMETRIC MEASUREMENTS

For anthropometric measurements, nutrition assessment includes the following:

- Classification of disease risk based on BMI (LD, HTN, DB, WM) [Table 2.8], where BMI is calculated as follows:
  - Weight (kg)/Height (m)^2
  - [Weight (lb)/Height (in)^2] × 703
- Classification of disease risk by WC (LD, DB, WM) [Table 2.8].

BMI and WC are also used in reassessment to determine the effectiveness of weight management therapy.

Table 2.8   Classification of Overweight and Obesity by Body Mass Index and Waist Circumference–Associated Disease Risk

Classification	BMI	WC-Associated Disease Risk[a]	
		≤WC Cutpoint[b]	>WC Cutpoint[c]
Underweight	<18.5		
Normal	18.5–24.9		Increased[d]
Overweight	25.0–29.9	Increased	High
Obesity (Class I)	30.0–34.9	High	Very high
Obesity (Class II)	35.0–39.9	Very high	Very high
Extreme obesity (Class III)	≥40	Extremely high	Extremely high

[a]Disease risk is for type 2 diabetes, hypertension, and CVD and compares with risk for an individual with normal BMI.
[b]WC cutpoint is defined for men as ≤40 inches (102 cm) and for women as ≤35 inches (88 cm). Lower WC cutpoints (≤35 inches [90 cm] in men and ≤31 inches [80 cm] in women) seem to be more appropriate for assessing increased disease risk in Asian Americans.
[c]WC cutpoint is defined for men as >40 inches (102 cm) and for women as >35 inches (88 cm).
[d]Even in persons of normal weight, WC can be associated with disease risk.
Source: Data are from references 17 and 35.

CLIENT HISTORY

It is essential to assess each client's relevant history, including the following factors (LD, HTN, DB, WM):

- Social history, such as socioeconomic status, occupation, social and medical support, cultural and religious beliefs, and housing situation
- Medical/health history and medical treatment, such as goals of medical therapy and prescribed medications related to the medical condition for which MNT is being implemented; the appropriateness of weight management
- Personal history factors (age, gender, role in family, education level, etc)
- Personal and family medical history
- Other medical treatments and complementary/alternative medicine

This section includes tables for use in nutrition assessment of medical history and medical treatments:

- Lipids (LD, HTN, DB, WM) [Table 2.9]
- Blood pressure (LD, HTN, DB, WM) [Table 2.10]
- Glycemia (DB)
  - Adults with diabetes [Table 2.11]
  - Type 1 diabetes by age groups [Table 2.12]
  - Correlation of A1C with average glucose [Table 2.13]
  - Gestational diabetes and preexisting type 1 or type 2 diabetes and pregnancy [Table 2.14]
- Weight management (WM, DB, LD, HTN) [Table 2.15]

Table 2.9   Lipid Treatment Guidelines

Finding	Treatment Goals and Therapies
Elevated LDL-C (>130 mg/dL [3.4 mmol/L])	• LDL-C goal: <100 mg/dL (2.6 mmol/L) (<70 mg/dL [1.8 mmol/L] for very high risk patients) • LDL-C ≥100 mg/dL (2.6 mmol/L): initiate lifestyle modifications (TLC[a]). • LDL-C ≥130 mg/dL (3.4 mmol/L): consider drug therapy.
Elevated TG (>200 mg/dL [2.3 mmol/L])	• Goal: TG <150 mg/dL (1.7 mmol/L) *or* non-HDL-C (total cholesterol – HDL) <130 mg/dL (3.4 mmol/L) • Primary aim of therapy is to reach LDL-C goal. • TG = 150–199 mg/dL (1.7–2.2 mmol/L): therapies are weight management and increased physical activity. • TG = 200–499 mg/dL (2.3–5.6 mmol/L): consider increasing dose of LDL-C drug to reach non-HDL-C goal (<130 mg/dL [2.6 mmol/L]) *or* add a fibrate or nicotinic acid to lower VLDL. • TG ≥500 mg/dL (5.7 mmol/L): first lower TG to prevent pancreatitis by initiating a very low-fat diet (<15% total kcal from fat), weight reduction, and increased physical activity; add fibrate or nicotinic acid.
Low HDL-C (<40 mg/dL [1.0 mmol/L] men, <50 mg/dL [1.3 mmol/L] women)	• First reach LDL-C goal, then intensify weight management and increase physical activity. • If TG are 200–499 mg/dL (2.3–5.6 mmol/L), achieve non-HDL goal. • If TG are <200 mg/dL (2.3 mmol/L) (isolated low HDL), consider adding fibrate or nicotinic acid.

[a]TLC intervention includes the following recommendations: saturated and *trans* fatty acids <7% of total energy intake; cholesterol intake <200 mg/day; weight reduction; and increased physical activity; also possibly consider increased soluble fiber (10–25 g/d) and use of plant stanols/sterols [2 g/d] to help lower LDL-C.
Source: Data are from reference 33.

Table 2.10 Blood Pressure Treatment Guidelines

Finding	Therapy Guidelines
BP <140/90 mmHg *or* BP <130/80 mmHg for individuals with diabetes or chronic kidney disease	• Lifestyle modification[a] • Initiate drug therapy
Stage 1 hypertension without compelling indications[b]	• Lifestyle modification[a] • Thiazide-type diuretics for most individuals • May consider ACEI, ARB, BB, CCB, or combination of these medications
Stage 2 hypertension without compelling indications[b]	• Lifestyle modification[a] • Two-drug combination for most (usually thiazide-type diuretic plus an ACEI or ARB or BB or CCB)
Hypertension with compelling indications[b]	• Lifestyle modification[a] • Other antihypertensive drugs (diuretics, ACEI, ARB, BB, CCB) as needed

Abbreviations: ACEI = angiotensin-converting enzyme inhibitor; ARB = angiotensin receptor blocker; BB = beta-blocker; CCB = calcium channel blocker.
[a]Lifestyle modification is defined as weight reduction, DASH eating plan, regular physical activity, and moderate alcohol intake.
[b]Compelling indications include heart failure, postmyocardial infarction, high coronary disease risk, diabetes, chronic kidney disease, or recurrent stroke prevention.
Source: Data are from reference 36.

Table 2.11   Management Goals for Adults with Diabetes

Glycemic control

- A1C <7%[a]
- Preprandial PG 70–130 mg/dL (3.9–7.2 mmol/L)
- Peak postprandial PG <180 mg/dL (10.0 mmol/L)

BP <130/80 mmHg

Lipids

- LDL-C <100 mg/dL[b] (2.6 mmol/L)
- TG <150 mg/dL (1.7 mmol/L)
- HDL-C:
  - >40 mg/dL (1.1 mmol/L) in men
  - >50 mg/dL (1.4 mmol/L) in women

[a]Referenced to a nondiabetic range of 4% to 6%, using a Diabetes Control and Complications Trial–based assay.

[b]In individuals with overt CVD, a lower LDL-C goal of <70 mg/dL (1.8 mmol/L) using a high dose of a statin, is an option.

Source: Adapted with permission from American Diabetes Association. Standards of medical care in diabetes—2010. *Diabetes Care.* 2010;33 (suppl 1):S11–S61. These data are also found in the reference 15: American Diabetes Association. Standards of medical care in diabetes—2012. *Diabetes Care*. 2012;35(suppl 1):S11–S63.

Table 2.12   Blood Glucose and A1C Goals for Youth with Type 1 Diabetes

Age Group (Ages, y)	Before-Meal PG Goal	Bedtime/ Overnight PG Goal	A1C
Toddlers and preschoolers (0–6)	100–180 mg/dL (5.6–10.0 mmol/L)	110–200 mg/dL (6.1–11.1 mmol/L)	<8.5 % (but >7.5%)
School age (6–12)	90–180 mg/dL (5.0–10.0 mmol/L)	100–180 mg/dL (5.6–10.0 mmol/L)	<8%
Adolescents and young adults (13–19)	90–130 mg/dL (5.0–7.2 mmol/L)	90–150 mg/dL (5.0–8.3 mmol/L)	<7.5%

Source: Adapted with permission from American Diabetes Association. Standards of medical care in diabetes—2010. *Diabetes Care.* 2010;33 (suppl 1):S11–S61. These data are also found in the reference 15: American Diabetes Association. Standards of medical care in diabetes—2012. *Diabetes Care*. 2012;35(suppl 1):S11–S63.

**Table 2.13   Correlation of A1C
with Mean Plasma Glucose**

	Mean Plasma Glucose	
A1C, %	*mg/dL*	*mmol/L*
6	126	7.0
7	154	8.6
8	183	10.2
9	212	11.8
10	240	13.4
11	269	14.9
12	298	16.5

Source: Reprinted with permission from American Diabetes Association. Standards of medical care in diabetes—2010. *Diabetes Care.* 2010;33 (suppl 1):S11–S61. These data are also found in the reference 15: American Diabetes Association. Standards of medical care in diabetes—2012. *Diabetes Care.* 2012;35 (suppl 1):S11–S63.

**Table 2.14   Plasma Glucose Goals for Pregnant Women
with GDM or Preexisting Type 1 or Type 2 Diabetes**

GDM
- Preprandial PG ≤95 mg/dL (5.3 mmol/L) and either:
  - 1-h postmeal PG ≤140 mg/dL (7.8 mmol/L) *or*
  - 2-h postmeal PG ≤120 mg/dL (6.7 mmol/L)

Preexisting type 1 or type 2 diabetes[a]
- Premeal, bedtime, and overnight PG 60–99 mg/dL (3.3–5.5 mmol/L)
- Peak postprandial PG 100–129 mg/dL (5.5–7.2 mmol/L)
- A1C <6%

[a]Recommend as optimal glycemic goals, if they can be achieved without excessive hypoglycemia.
Source: Adapted from with permission from American Diabetes Association. Standards of medical care in diabetes—2010. *Diabetes Care.* 2010;33(suppl 1):S11–S61. These data are also found in the reference 15: American Diabetes Association. Standards of medical care in diabetes—2012. *Diabetes Care.* 2012;35 (suppl 1):S11–S63.

Table 2.15   Energy Requirement Calculations in Overweight and Obesity

---

TEE = RMR × Physical Activity Factor

Estimating RMR in overweight/obese individuals:

If indirect calorimetry is not available, use the Mifflin-St. Jeor equation:

Men: RMR = $(10 \times$ Weight$) + (6.25 \times$ Height$) - (5 \times$ Age$) + 5$

Women: RMR = $(10 \times$ Weight$) + (6.25 \times$ Height$) - (5 \times$ Age$) - 161$

Where: Weight is actual weight (kg); height is measured in cm and age in years.

Selecting a physical activity factor:

Use clinical judgment to determine the physical activity component of the individual's TEE. Definitions for physical activity determinations are in parentheses.

DRI Physical Activity Factors:

- **≥1 to <1.4: Sedentary** (reflects basal metabolism, thermic effect of food, and physical activities required for independent living)
- **≥1.4 to <1.6: Low active** (same as sedentary plus daily physical activity equivalent to walking approximately 2 miles/d at 15 to 20 min/mile *or* an equivalent amount of other moderate-intensity activities—such as golfing without a cart, raking leaves, vigorous housework or gardening, or taking a low-impact aerobics class—each day)
- **≥1.6 to <1.9: Active** (same as sedentary plus daily physical activity equivalent to approximately 105 minutes of moderate-intensity activities *or* 70 minutes of vigorous-intensity activities, such as bicycle riding, tennis, or jogging)
- **≥1.9 to <2.5: Very active** (same as sedentary plus daily physical activity equivalent to approximately 250 minutes of moderate-intensity physical activities *or* 160 minutes of vigorous-intensity activities)

Source: Adapted with permission from reference 37: American Dietetic Association. *Adult Weight Management Toolkit.* Chicago, IL, American Dietetic Association; 2007.

FOOD-/NUTRITION-RELATED HISTORY

Food-/nutrition-related history nutrition assessment includes the following (LD, HTN, DB, WM):

- Energy intake
- Macronutrient intake
- Readiness to change nutrition-related behaviors, using the transtheoretical model of intentional change (Stages of Change) (see Chapter 5)
- Behavioral factors that influence achievement of nutrition-related goals
- History of previous nutrition care services/MNT
- Physical activity
  - **Note**: Energy expenditure in physical activity can be estimated by either of two methods: (*a*) using tables that list physical activities and kilocalories expended per hour based on body weight; or (*b*) determining energy spent by adults during various intensities of physical activity—energy that is expressed as metabolic equivalents (METs), units of measure that correspond to an individual's metabolic rate during physical activities of varying intensities and are expressed as multiples of resting metabolic rates. A MET value of 1 is the oxygen metabolized at rest and is 1 kcal per kg of body weight per hour. For example, an individual walking at a very brisk pace (4 mph) expends 5 METs which is 5 times the energy he or she would expend at rest.
- Other medications (ie, those not prescribed for MNT-related condition) and complementary/alternative medicine use

The remaining tables in this chapter aid in the assessment of physical activity [Tables 2.16–2.20] and medication use [Tables 2.21–2.43].

Table 2.16   Physical Activity Guidelines

Adults

- Engage in 2½ hours of moderate-intensity aerobic physical activity[a] or 1¼ hours of vigorous-intensity physical activity[b] per week.
- Aerobic activity should be performed in episodes at least 10 minutes in duration.
- For more extensive health benefits, increase aerobic physical activity to 5 hours of moderate-intensity or 2½ hours of vigorous-intensity physical activity per week.
- Incorporate muscle-strengthening activities[c] at least 2 days per week.

Older adults

- When physically capable, follow the guidelines for other adults.
- If older adults have a chronic condition that prohibits their ability to follow guidelines, they should be as physically active as abilities and conditions allow.
- If older adults are at risk of falling, they should do exercises to maintain and improve balance.

Women during pregnancy

- During pregnancy and the time after delivery, do 2½ hours of moderate-intensity aerobic activity[a] per week, with activity preferably spread throughout the week.
- Women who habitually engage in vigorous-intensity aerobic activity[b] or are highly active before pregnancy can continue activities during pregnancy and the time after delivery, provided they remain healthy and discuss with their health care provider how and when activity should be adjusted over time.

Adults with disabilities

- If able, do 2½ hours of moderate-intensity aerobic activity[a] or 1¼ hours of vigorous-intensity activity[b] per week.
- Incorporate muscle-strengthening activities[c] involving all major groups at least 2 days per week.
- If adults are not able to meet these guidelines, they should engage in regular physical activity according to their abilities and avoid inactivity.

People with chronic medical conditions

- Seek the important health benefits of regular physical activity under the guidance of a health care provider.

(continues on next page)

Table 2.16 **Physical Activity Guidelines** (continued)

Children and adolescents

- Aim for at least 1 hour of moderate-intensity[a] or vigorous-intensity[b] aerobic physical activity daily, including vigorous-intensity activities at least 3 days per week.
- Include muscle-strengthening[c] and bone-strengthening[d] activities 3 days per week.

[a]Moderate-intensity activities for adults include walking briskly, water aerobics, ballroom dancing, and general gardening. Examples for children and adolescents include hiking, skateboarding, bicycle riding, and brisk walking.
[b]Vigorous-intensity activities for adults include race walking, jogging or running, swimming laps, jumping rope, or hiking uphill or with a heavy backpack. Examples for children and adolescents include bicycle riding, jumping rope, running, and sports such as soccer, basketball, and ice or field hockey.
[c]Muscle-strengthening activities for adults include weight training, push-ups, sit-ups, and carrying heavy loads or heavy gardening. Examples for children and adolescents include rope climbing, sit-ups, and tug-of-war.
[d]Bone-strengthening activities for children and adolescents include jumping rope, running, and skipping.
Source: Data are from reference 18.

Table 2.17 **Physical Activity (PA) Intervention Strategies for Weight Control in Adults**

Goal	Physical Activity Strategy
Prevention of weight gain	• 150–250 min PA per week (1,200–1,500 kcal/wk) prevents weight gain greater than 3% in most adults.
Weight loss	• PA <150 min/wk promotes minimal weight loss. • PA >150 min/wk results in modest weight loss (~2–3 kg). • PA >225–420 min/wk results in 5–7.5 kg weight loss, and a dose-response exists.
Weight maintenance after weight loss	• During weight maintenance, a minimum of approximately 200–300 minutes PA per week may reduce weight regain after weight loss; however, more PA is better.

Source: Data are from reference 19.

**Table 2.18   Metabolic Equivalents of Common Light
(<3 METs) Physical Activities**[a]

Activity	METs
Arts and crafts	1.5
Billiards	2.5
Croquet	2.5
Darts	2.5
Fishing (sitting)	2.5
Light housework performed standing, such as making beds, washing dishes, ironing, or preparing food	2.0–2.5
Playing cards	1.5
Playing most musical instruments	2.0–2.5
Power boating	2.5
Sitting and using computer or working at desk, using light hand tools	1.5
Walking slowly around home, store or office	2.0
Working as a store clerk (standing)	2.0–2.5

[a]MET = metabolic equivalent. One MET represents an individual's energy expenditure while sitting quietly.
Source: Data are from reference 38.

Table 2.19   Metabolic Equivalents of Common Moderate (3–6 METs) Physical Activities[a]

Activity	METs
Badminton, recreational	4.5
Basketball—shooting around	4.5
Bicycling on flat terrain; light effort (10–12 mph)	6.0
Carpentry, general	3.6
Carrying and stacking wood	5.5
Cleaning garage	3.0
Dancing, fast ballroom	4.5
Dancing, slow ballroom	3.0
Fishing from river bank and walking	4.0
Golf—walking and pulling clubs	4.3
Mopping	3.0–3.5
Mowing lawn with walk power mower	5.5
Sailing	3.0
Sweeping floors or carpet	3.0–3.5
Swimming leisurely	6.0
Table tennis	4.0
Tennis doubles	5.0
Vacuuming	3.0–3.5
Volleyball, noncompetitive	3.0–4.0
Walking 3.0 mph	3.3
Walking at very brisk pace (4 mph)	5.0
Washing windows or car	3.0
Wind surfing	3.0

[a]MET = metabolic equivalent. One MET represents an individual's energy expenditure while sitting quietly.
Source: Data are from reference 38.

Table 2.20   Metabolic Equivalents of Common Vigorous (>6.0 METs) Physical Activities[a]

Activity	METs
Basketball game	8.0
Bicycling fast (14–16 mph)	10.0
Bicycling on flat terrain; moderate effort (12–14 mph)	8.0
Carrying heavy loads (such as bricks)	7.5
Digging ditches	8.5
Heavy farming (such as baling hay)	8.0
Hiking at steep grades and pack (10–42 lb)	7.5–9.0
Jogging at 5 mph	8.0
Jogging at 6 mph	10.0
Running at 7 mph	11.5
Shoveling	8.5
Shoveling (sand, coal, etc)	7.0
Skiing cross country, fast (5.0–7.9 mph)	9.0
Skiing cross country, slow (2.5 mph)	7.0
Soccer, casual	7.0
Soccer, competitive	10.0
Swimming, moderate/hard	8.0–11.0
Tennis, singles	8.0
Volleyball, competitive at gym or beach	8.0
Walking at very, very brisk pace (4.5 mph)	6.3
Walking/hiking at moderate pace and grade with no or light pack (<10 lb)	7.0

[a]MET = metabolic equivalent. One MET represents an individual's energy expenditure while sitting quietly.
Source: Data are from reference 38.

Table 2.21 Types of Lipid-Lowering Agents: HMG CoA Reductase Inhibitors (Statins)

Agent (Brand Name)	Daily Dosage
Atorvastatin (Lipitor)	10–80 mg
Fluvastatin (Lescol)	20–80 mg
Fluvastatin, extended release (Lescol XL)	80 mg
Lovastatin (Mevacor)	20–80 mg
Lovastatin, extended release (Altocor)	10–60 mg
Pravastatin (Pravachol)	20–40 mg
Rosuvastatin (Crestor)	10–40 mg
Simvastatin (Zocor)	20–80 mg

Source: Data are from reference 33.

Table 2.22 Types of Lipid-Lowering Agents: Fibrates (Fibric Acids)

Agent (Brand Name)	Daily Dosage
Clofibrate (Atromid-S)	1,000 mg twice daily
Fenofibrate (TriCor)	200 mg
Fenofibric acid (Trilipix)	45–135 mg
Gemfibrozil (Lopid)	600 mg twice daily

Source: Data are from reference 33.

Table 2.23 Types of Lipid-Lowering Agents: Bile Acid Sequestrants (Binding Resins)

Agent (Brand Name)	Daily Dosage
Cholestyramine (Questran, Questran Light)	4–16 g
Colesevelam (Welchol)	2.6–3.8 g
Colestipol (Colestid)	5–20 g

Source: Data are from reference 33.

Table 2.24   Types of Lipid-Lowering Agents:
Cholesterol Absorption Inhibitors, Niacin, and Fish Oils

Agent (Brand Name)	Daily Dosage
Ezetimibe (Zetia)[a]	10 mg
Niacin/nicotinic acid	1.5–3 g
Niacin, extended release (Niaspan)	1–2 g
Omega-3-acid ethyl esters (Lovaza)[b]	4 g

[a]Cholesterol absorption inhibitor.
[b]A lipid-regulating agent for patients with severe hypertriglyceridemia (TG ≥500 mg/dL [5.7 mmol/L]); not included in reference 33.
Source: Data are from reference 33.

Table 2.25   Types of Lipid-Lowering Agents:
Combination Agents

Agent (Brand Name)	Daily Dosage
Niacin, extended release/lovastatin (Advicor)	1–2 tabs
Atorvastatin/norvasc (Caduet)	1 tab
Ezetimibe/simvastatin (Vytorin)	1 tab

Source: Data are from reference 33.

Table 2.26 Effects of Lipid-Lowering Agents

Drug Class	Lipid/Lipoprotein Effects
HMG CoA reductase inhibitors (statins)	LDL-C ↓ 18%–55% HDL-C ↑ 5%–15% TG ↓ 7%–30%
Fibrates (fibric acids)	LDL-C ↓ 5%–20% (may be increased in individuals with high TG) HDL-C ↑ 10%–20% TG ↓ 20%–50%
Bile acid sequestrants (binding resins)	LDL-C ↓ 15%–30% HDL ↑ 3%–5% TG No change
Cholesterol absorption inhibitors	LDL-C ↓ 18% TG ↓ 8% Apo B ↓ 16%
Niacin (nicotinic acid)	LDL-C ↓ 5%–25% HDL-C ↑ 15%–35% TG ↓ 20%–50%
Lipid-regulating agent (fish oils)[a]	TG ↓ 45% LDL-C ↑ in some individuals

[a]A lipid-regulating agent for patients with severe hypertriglyceridemia (TG ≥500 mg/dL); not included in reference 33.
Source: Data are from reference 33.

Table 2.27   Oral Antihypertensive Drugs: Thiazide Diuretics

Drug (Brand Name)	Usual Daily Dosing Range (Daily Frequency)
Chlorothiazide (Diuril)	125–500 mg (once)
Hydrochlorothiazide (Microzide, HydroDIURIL)	12.5–50 mg (once)
Indapamide (Lozol)	1.25–2.5 mg (once)
Metolazone (Mykrox)	0.5–1.0 mg (once)
Metolazone (Zaroxolyn)	2.5–5 mg (once)
Polythiazide (Renese)	2–4 mg (once)

Source: Data are from reference 36.

Table 2.28   Oral Antihypertensive Drugs: Loop Diuretics

Drug (Brand Name)	Usual Daily Dosing Range (Daily Frequency)
Bumetanide (Bumex)	0.5–2 mg (twice)
Furosemide (Lasix)	20–80 mg (twice)
Torsemide (Dyrenium)	2.5–10 mg (once)

Source: Data are from reference 36.

Table 2.29   Oral Antihypertensive Drugs: Potassium-Sparing Diuretics

Drug (Brand Name)	Usual Daily Dosing Range (Daily Frequency)
Amiloride (Midamor)	5–10 mg (once or twice)
Triamterene (Dyrenium)	50–100 mg (once to twice)

Source: Data are from reference 36.

Table 2.30   Oral Antihypertensive Drugs: Aldosterone Receptor Blockers

Drug (Brand Name)	Usual Daily Dosing Range (Daily Frequency)
Eplerenone (Inspra)	50–100 mg (once or twice)
Spironolactone (Aldactone)	25–50 mg (once or twice)

Source: Data are from reference 36.

Table 2.31   Oral Antihypertensive Drugs: Beta-Blockers

Drug (Brand Name)	Usual Daily Dosing Range (Daily Frequency)
Atenolol (Tenormin)	25–100 mg (once)
Betaxolol (Kerlone)	5–20 mg (once)
Bisoprolol (Zebeta)	2.5–10 mg (once)
Metoprolol (Lopressor)	50–100 mg (once or twice)
Metoprolol extended release (Toprol XL)	50–100 mg (once)
Nadolol (Corgard)	40–120 mg (once)
Propranolol (Inderal)	40–160 mg (twice)
Propranolol long-acting (Inderal LA)	60–180 mg (once)
Timolol (Blocadren)	20–40 mg (twice)

Source: Data are from reference 36.

Table 2.32   Oral Antihypertensive Drugs: Beta-Blockers with Intrinsic Sympathomimetic Activity

Drug (Brand Name)	Usual Daily Dosing Range (Daily Frequency)
Acebutolol (Sectral)	200–800 mg (twice)
Penbutolol (Levatol)	10–40 mg (once)

Source: Data are from reference 36.

Table 2.33   Oral Antihypertensive Drugs: Combined Alpha- and Beta-Blockers

Drug (Brand Name)	Usual Daily Dosing Range (Daily Frequency)
Carvedilol (Coreg)	12.5–50 mg (twice)
Labetalol (Normodyne, Trandate)	200–800 mg (twice)

Source: Data are from reference 36.

Table 2.34   Oral Antihypertensive Drugs: ACE Inhibitors

Drug (Brand Name)	Usual Daily Dosing Range (Daily Frequency)
Benazepril (Lotensin)	10–40 mg (once or twice)
Captopril (Capoten)	25–100 mg (twice)
Enalapril (Vasotec)	2.5–40 mg (once or twice)
Fosinopril (Monopril)	10–40 mg (once)
Lisinopril (Prinivil, Zestril)	10–40 mg (once)
Moexipril (Univasc)	7.5–30 mg (once)
Perindopril (Aceon)	4–8 mg (once or twice)
Quinapril (Accupril)	10–40 mg (once)
Ramipril (Altace)	2.5–20 mg (once)
Trandolapril (Mavik)	1–4 mg (once)

Source: Data are from reference 36.

Table 2.35 Oral Antihypertensive Drugs: Angiotensin II Antagonists

Drug (Brand Name)	Usual Daily Dosing Range (Daily Frequency)
Candesartan (Atacand)	8–32 mg (once)
Eprosartan (Tevetan)	400–800 mg (once or twice)
Irbesartan (Avapro)	150–300 mg (once)
Losartan (Cozaar)	25–100 mg (once or twice)
Olmesartan (Benicar)	20–40 mg (once)
Telmisartan (Micardis)	20–80 mg (once)
Valsartan (Diovan)	80–320 mg (once)

Source: Data are from reference 36.

Table 2.36 Oral Antihypertensive Drugs: Calcium Channel Blockers—Non-Dihydropyridines

Drug (Brand Name)	Usual Daily Dosing Range (Daily Frequency)
Diltiazem extended release (Cardizem CD, Dilacor XR, Tiazac)	180–420 mg (once)
Diltiazem extended release (Cardizem LA)	120–540 mg (once)
Verapamil immediate release (Calan, Isoptin)	80–320 mg (twice)
Verapamil long acting (Calan SR, Isoptin SR)	120–360 mg (once or twice)
Verapamil-Coer (Covera HS, Verelan PM)	120–360 mg (once)

Source: Data are from reference 36.

**Table 2.37 Oral Antihypertensive Drugs:
Calcium Channel Blockers—Dihydropyridines**

Drug (Brand Name)	Usual Daily Dosing Range (Daily Frequency)
Amlodipine (Norvasc)	2.5–10 mg (once)
Felodipine (Plendil)	2.5–20 mg (once)
Isradipine (Dynacirc CR)	2.5–10 mg (once)
Nicardipine sustained release (Cardene SR)	60–120 mg (twice)
Nifedipine long-acting (Adalat CC, Procardia XL)	30–60 mg (once)
Nisoldipine (Sular)	10–40 mg (once)

Source: Data are from reference 36.

Table 2.38 Oral Antihypertensive Drugs: Alpha$_1$-Blockers

Drug (Brand Name)	Usual Daily Dosing Range (Daily Frequency)
Doxazosin (Cardura)	1–16 mg (once)
Prazosin (Minipress)	2–20 mg (twice or three)
Terazosin (Hytrin)	1–20 mg (once or twice)

Source: Data are from reference 36.

Table 2.39 Oral Antihypertensive Drugs: Central Alpha₂-Agonists and Other Centrally Acting Drugs

Drug (Brand Name)	Usual Daily Dosing Range (Daily Frequency)
Clonidine (Catapres)	0.1–0.8 mg (twice)
Clonidine patch (Catapres-TTS)	0.1–0.3 mg (once/wk)
Methyldopa (Aldomet)	250–1,000 mg (twice)
Reserpine (generic)	0.05–0.25 mg (once)
Guanfacine (generic)	0.5–2 mg (once)

Source: Data are from reference 36.

Table 2.40 Oral Antihypertensive Drugs: Direct Vasodilators

Drug (Brand Name)	Usual Daily Dosing Range (Daily Frequency)
Hydralazine (Apresoline)	25–100 mg (twice)
Minoxidil (Loniten)	2.5–80 mg (once or twice)

Source: Data are from reference 36.

Table 2.41   Glucose-Lowering Medications for Type 2 Diabetes

Biguanide class
- Examples: Metformin (Glucophage and Glucophage XR)
- Expected decrease in A1C with monotherapy (unit decrease): 1%–2%
- Principal action: Decrease hepatic glucose production
- Advantages: Weight neutral; minimal hypoglycemia; lipid neutral; relatively inexpensive
- Disadvantages: GI upset
- Usual dosage information:
  - Glucophage: 500 mg/d twice a day with meals, increase by 500 mg every 1–3 wk, twice or three times a day; usually most effective at 2,000 mg/d; maximum 2,550 mg/d
  - Glucophage XR: 500 mg once a day; maximum 2,000 mg once a day

Sulfonylureas (second generation)
- Examples:
  - Glipizide (Glucotrol and Glucotrol XL)
  - Glyburide (Glynase Prestabs)
  - Glimepiride (Amaryl)
- Expected decrease in A1C with mono-therapy (unit decrease): 1%–2%
- Principal action: Stimulate insulin action from the beta cell of the pancreas
- Advantages: Inexpensive; effective in combination; been used for years
- Disadvantages: Hypoglycemia; weight gain; loss of response with time
- Usual dosage information:
  - Glucotrol: 2.5–20 mg once or twice a day; maximum 40 mg/d
  - Glucotrol XL: 2.5–10 mg once or twice day; maximum 20 mg/d
  - Glynase: 1.5–3 to 12 mg/d; maximum 12 mg/d
  - Amaryl: 1–8 mg/d; maximum 8 mg/d

Thiazolidinediones
- Examples:
  - Rosiglitazone (Avandia)
  - Pioglitazone (Actos; note warnings on label regarding increased risk of cancer)
- Expected decrease in A1C with mono-therapy (unit decrease): 0.5%–1.4%
- Principal action: Improve peripheral insulin sensitivity
- Advantages: Improved lipid profile (pioglitazone); no hypoglycemia
- Disadvantages: Weight gain; fluid retention; CHF; bone fractures; requires liver function monitoring; potential increase in MI (rosiglitazone); expensive

(continues on next page)

Table 2.41   Glucose-Lowering Medications for Type 2 Diabetes
(continued)

- Usual dosage information:
  - Actos: initially 15 or 30 mg/d; maximum (with or without food) 45 mg/d for monotherapy, 30 mg/d for combination therapy
  - Avandia: initially 4 mg/d in single or divided doses; increase to 8 mg/d in 12 weeks, if needed; maximum (with or without food) 8 mg/d

Glucagon-like peptide-1 (GLP-1) agonist
- Examples:
  - Exantide (Byetta, Bydureon)
  - Liraglutide (Victoza)
- Expected decrease in A1C with mono-therapy (unit decrease): 0.5%–1.5%
- Principal action: Potentiates glucose-stimulated insulin secretion, suppresses glucagon release, and slows gastric emptying
- Advantages: Weight loss; no hypoglycemia
- Disadvantages: Byetta two injections daily and Victoza one injection daily; frequent GI adverse effects (initially, dosing immediately before meals reduces nausea, with time, increase to 30–60 min); long-term safety not established; expensive
- Usual dosage information:
  - Byetta: initially 5 mcg within 60 minutes of morning and evening meals (never after meal); titrate to 10 mcg twice a day after 1 month based on tolerability and glycemic control
  - Bydureon: once weekly, extended-release formulation of exenatide injection
  - Victoza: once daily at any time, independently of meals; initially 0.6 mg/day for 1 week, then increase to 1.2 mg/d; maximum dose 1.8 mg/d

Alpha glucosidase inhibitors
- Examples:
  - Acarbose (Precose)
  - Miglitol (Glyset)
- Expected decrease in A1C with monotherapy (unit decrease): 0.5%–0.8%
- Principal action: delay carbohydrate absorption
- Advantages: Low systemic toxicity; reduce postprandial glucose; no weight gain
- Disadvantages: Poorly tolerated due to flatulence and diarrhea; expensive

(continues on next page)

Table 2.41   Glucose-Lowering Medications for Type 2 Diabetes
(continued)

- Disadvantages: Poorly tolerated due to flatulence and diarrhea; expensive
- Usual dosage information:
  - Precose: 25 mg/d, increase by 25 mg/d every 4–6 weeks; maximum 300 mg/d, split dose before meals (with first bite of food)
  - Glyset: 300 mg/d (150 mg/d for individuals weighing <60 kg)

Glinides
- Examples:
  - Repaglinide (Prandin)
  - Nateglinide (Starlix)
- Expected decrease in A1C with monotherapy (unit decrease): 0.5%–1.5%
- Principal action: Stimulate insulin secretion from the beta cells of the pancreas
- Advantages: Used before meals and short-acting; lower risk of hypoglycemia than with sulfonylureas; can be used in renal insufficiency
- Disadvantages: Must be taken before meals (multiple dosing); less effective with prior sulfonylurea failure
- Usual dosage information:
  - Prandin: new diagnosis or A1C <8%, 0.5 mg, 15–30 minutes before each meal; A1C >8%, 1–2 mg, 15–30 minutes before each meal; increase dosage weekly until results are obtained; maximum 16 mg/d
  - Starlix: 60–120 mg before each meal

Amylin agonists
- Example: Pramlintide (Symlin)
- Expected decrease in A1C with mono-therapy (unit decrease): 0.5–1.0%
- Principal action: Inhibits glucagon release in a glucose-dependent manner and slows gastric emptying; indicated for insulin-treated type 2 diabetes or for type 1 diabetes
- Advantages: Weight loss; decreases postprandial glucose excursions
- Disadvantages: Three injections daily; frequent side effects (GI); long-term safety not established; expensive

(continues on next page)

Table 2.41   Glucose-Lowering Medications for Type 2 Diabetes
(continued)

- Usual dosage information:
  - Type 1 diabetes: 15–60 mcg per meal starting with 15 mcg before meals of 30 g or more carbohydrate
  - Type 2 diabetes: 60–120 mcg per meal starting with 60 mcg before meals

Dipeptidyl peptidase-4 (DPP-4) inhibitors
- Examples:
  - Sitagliptin (Januvia)
  - Saxagliptin (Onglyza)
  - Linagliptin (Tradjenta)
  - Vildagliptin (Galvus)
- Expected decrease in A1C with monotherapy (unit decrease): 0.5%–0.8%
- Principal action: Enhance the effects of GLP-1 and GIP by preventing degradation
- Advantages: Weight neutral; well tolerated; do not cause hypoglycemia when used as monotherapy
- Disadvantages: Long-term safety not established; expensive
- Usual dosage information:
  - Januvia: 100 mg once daily with or without food
  - Onglyza: 5 mg once daily

Bile acid sequestrants
- Example: Colesevelam (Welchol)
- Principal action: Binds bile acids/cholesterol
- Advantages: No hypoglycemia; lowers LDL cholesterol
- Disadvantages: Constipation, increased triglycerides; may interfere with absorption of other medications

Dopamine-2 agonists
- Example: Bromocriptine (Cycloset)
- Principal action: Activates dopaminergic receptors
- Advantages: No hypoglycemia
- Disadvantages: Dizziness/syncope, nausea, fatigue, rhinitis; long-term safety unknown

Source: Data are from reference 15: American Diabetes Association. Standards of medical care—2012. *Diabetes Care*. 2012;35(suppl 1):S11–264.

Table 2.42 Insulins

Type (Brand Name)	Onset of Action	Peak Action	Usual Effective Duration	Monitor Effect in
Rapid-acting				
Lispro (Humalog)	<0.25–0.5 h	0.5–2.5 h	3–6.5 h	1–2 h
Aspart (Novolog)	<0.25 h	0.5–1.0 h	3–5 h	1–2 h
Glulisine (Apidra)	<0.25	1–1.5 h	3–5 h	1–2 h
Short-acting				
Regular (Humulin R and Novolin R)	0.5–1 h	2–3 h	3–6 h	4 h (next meal)
Intermediate-acting				
NPH	2–4 h	4–10 h	10–16 h	8–12 h
Long-acting				
Glargine (Lantus)	2–4	Relatively flat	20–24 h	10–12 h

(continues on next page)

Table 2.42 Insulins (continued)

Type (Brand Name)	Onset of Action	Peak Action	Usual Effective Duration	Monitor Effect in
Long-acting				
Determir (Levemir)	0.8–2 h (dose dependent)	Relatively flat	Dose dependent: 12 h for 0.2 U/kg; 20 h for 0.4 U/kg; up to 24 h	10–12 h
Mixtures				
70/30[a]	0.5–1 h	Dual	10–16 h	
Humalog Mix 75/25[b]	<0.25 h	Dual	10–16 h	
Humalog Mix 50/50[c]	<0.25 h	Dual	10–16 h	
Novolog Mix 70/30[d]	<0.25 h	Dual	10–16 h	

[a]70% NPH, 30% ie regular.   [b]75% neutral protamine lispro (NPL), 25% lispro.
[c]50% NPL, 50% lispro.   [d]70% neutral protamine aspart (NPA), 30% aspart.

Source: Adapted with permission from reference 39: Kaufman FR, ed. *Medical Management of Type 1 Diabetes.* 5th ed. Alexandria, VA: American Diabetes Association; 2008.

Table 2.43   Pharmacological Therapy for Obesity

Orlistat
- Brand names: Xenical (120 mg); Alli (over-the-counter; 60 mg).
- Description: An intestinal fat absorption inhibitor that inhibits gastrointestinal lipases.
- Dosage: Xenical: 120 mg twice daily with meals; Alli: 60 mg taken during or within 1 hour after a meal containing some fat (no more than 30% of meal calories from fat), usually taken three times daily.
- Adverse effects include diarrhea and greasy stools.

Weight loss drugs under investigation:
- *Qnexa* (developed by Vivus Inc) is a combination of phentermine and controlled-release topiramate. Adverse effects include an increase in heart rate to 1 to 2 beats per minute and a two- to fivefold increased risk of cleft lip among children born to women taking topiramate. The FDA Drug Advisory Committee voted in favor of approving Qnexa in February 2012. FDA will make a decision in July 2012.
- *Lorcaserin* (developed by Arena Pharmaceutical) is a novel single agent that represents the first in a new class of selective serotonin 2 C receptor agonists that resulted in 5% or more weight loss plus improvements in secondary endpoints associated with cardiovascular risk. The company is in the process of trying to obtain FDA approval for the drug (brand name Lorquess). Studies reported a smaller weight loss compared with other weight-loss drugs.
- *Contrave* (developed by Orexigen Therapeutics) is a combination of two medications, bupropion SR and naltrexone SR, that in phase 3 trials resulted in weight loss of at least 5% after 56 weeks and improvements in secondary endpoints such as waist circumference, visceral fat, HDL-C, and TG. The company is in the process of trying to obtain FDA approval for the drug.

Source: Data are from reference 29.

Chapter 3

Nutrition Diagnosis

The nutrition diagnosis identifies and describes a specific nutrition problem that can be resolved or improved through treatment or intervention by an RD. The nutrition diagnosis is derived from the findings from the nutrition assessment and the RD's clinical judgment, and it is used as the basis for determining the nutrition prescription and nutrition interventions, including the nutrition-related goals (for more on the nutrition intervention step, see Chapters 4 and 5).

Nutrition diagnoses are not medical diagnoses. They are actual or predicted nutrition-related problems. To accurately determine nutrition diagnoses, the RD reviews the client/patient's symptoms and compares them to the signs and symptoms in the *International Dietetics & Nutrition Terminology (IDNT) Reference Manual: Standardized Language for the Nutrition Care Process* (2). Clients/patients may have more than one nutrition diagnosis, in which case the RD will need to prioritize the diagnoses in the nutrition intervention step.

The IDNT organizes nutrition diagnoses in the following four categories (2):

- **Intake**: defined as "actual problems related to intake of energy, nutrients, fluids, bioactive substances through oral diet or nutrition support."
- **Clinical**: defined as "nutritional findings/problems identified that relate to medical or physical conditions."

- **Behavioral-Environmental**: defined as "nutritional findings/problems identified that relate to knowledge, attitudes/beliefs, physical environment, access to food, or food safety."
- **Other**: defined as "nutrition findings that are not classified as intake, clinical, or behavioral-environmental problems."

Once a nutrition problem or diagnosis has been described, the RD identifies the etiology of the problem so that recommendations for nutrition intervention(s) focus on eliminating the cause or contributing risk factors. Each nutrition diagnosis is written in a PES (problem, etiology, signs and symptoms) format. The PES statement describes the problem, its root cause, and the assessment data that support the nutrition diagnosis.

POSSIBLE NUTRITION DIAGNOSES AND EXAMPLES OF PES STATEMENTS

The following sections feature possible nutrition diagnoses and sample PES statements. These examples might be used by RDs for implementation of nutrition therapy for lipid disorders, hypertension, diabetes, and weight management.

The particular EBNPG to which the nutrition diagnosis and PES statements apply are noted in the parentheses using this key:

- **LD** = lipid disorders
- **HTN** = hypertension
- **DB** = diabetes
- **WM** = weight management

Other abbreviations are listed on pages xi–xiii.

Intake

Nutrition Diagnosis: Less than optimal intake of types of fats (LD, DB, HTN, WM)

Sample PES Statement: Excessive saturated fat intake (P) related to lack of knowledge of saturated fat content of foods (E) as evidenced by self-report of high saturated fat intake and elevated laboratory values: TC = 300 mg/dL, LDL-C = 165 mg/dL (S).

Nutrition Diagnosis: Excessive energy intake (LD, HTN, DB, WM)

Sample PES Statement: Excessive energy intake (P) related to food and knowledge deficit (E) as evidenced by self-reported food intake and limited physical activity level as well as changing anthropometrics: 10-pound weight gain in 3 months, BMI = 27 (S).

Sample PES Statement: Excessive energy intake (P) related to frequent consumption of large portions of high-fat meals (E) as evidenced by average daily energy intake that exceeds recommended amount by 500 kcal and 12-pound weight gain during the past 18 months (S).

Nutrition Diagnosis: Excessive mineral intake (HTN, LD, DB, WM)

Sample PES Statement: Excessive sodium intake (P) related to overconsumption of fast-food meals and pre-packaged foods (E) as evidenced by food history that indicates more than 4-grams of sodium consumed daily as well as recent increase in blood pressure to 140/90 mmHg (S).

Nutrition Diagnosis: Inconsistent carbohydrate intake (DB)

Sample PES Statement: Inconsistent carbohydrate intake (P) related to incorrect application of carbohydrate counting to diabetes management (E) as evidenced by food records revealing two additional carbohydrate servings per meals and elevated fasting blood glucose levels of 155–210 mg/dL most days of the week (S).

Sample PES Statement: Inconsistent carbohydrate intake (P) related to inability to modify eating pattern when work schedule changes (E) as evidenced by fluctuations in blood glucose level and eating only one large meal daily (S).

Nutrition Diagnosis: Less than optimal intake of types of carbohydrate (DB, LD, WM)

Sample PES Statement: Excessive intake of sugars (P) related to food and knowledge deficit (E) as evidenced by frequent self-reported intake of regular soft drinks (S).

Nutrition Diagnosis: Excessive carbohydrate intake (DB, WM)

Sample PES Statement: Excessive carbohydrate intake relative to insulin dosing (P) related to inaccurate carbohydrate counting (E) as evidenced by the number of carbohydrate servings per meal noted in food record as well as postmeal blood glucose consistently >200 mg/dL (S).

Nutrition Diagnosis: Excessive alcohol intake (WM, LD, DB, HTN)

Sample PES Statement: Excessive alcohol intake (P) related to lack of knowledge on value for limiting intake (E) as evidenced by drinking 4 to 5 beers daily and patient reports of no interest in changing intake (S).

Clinical

Nutrition Diagnosis: Altered nutrition-related laboratory values (LD, DB, HTN)

Sample PES Statement: Abnormal LDL-C values (P) related to high saturated fat intake from food (E) as evidenced by elevated LDL-C of 165 mg/dL and food history that indicates >10% of energy intake is from saturated fats (S).

Sample PES Statement: Altered blood glucose values (P) related to insufficient insulin (E) as evidenced by hyperglycemia despite very good eating habits (S).

Nutrition Diagnosis: Overweight/obesity (LD, HTN, DB, WM)

Sample PES Statement: Overweight (P) related to excessive energy intake with limited physical activity (E) as evidenced by BMI of 30 and lifestyle history that indicates a sedentary lifestyle and consumption of 2,800 kcal/d vs estimated needs of 2,200 kcal/d (S).

Nutrition Diagnosis: Unintended weight loss (DB)

Sample PES Statement: Unintended weight loss (P) related to inadequate insulin due to type 1 diabetes (E) as evidenced by rapid 15-pound weight loss during the past several weeks and elevated A1C of 10% (S).

Nutrition Diagnosis: Impaired nutrient utilization (DB)

Sample PES Statement: Impaired nutrient utilization (P) related to type 2 (or type 1) diabetes (E) as evidenced by elevated postmeal glucose levels even when patient eats recommended carbohydrate servings at meals and snacks (S).

Nutrition Diagnosis: Food-medication interaction (LD, HTN, DB, WM)

Sample PES Statement: Food-medication interaction (P) related to fluctuating vitamin K intake while on warfarin (E) as evidenced by food history suggesting wide fluctuation in intake of dark greens and lab results indicating that international normalized ratio (INR) is not within recommended level (S).

Behavioral-Environmental

Nutrition Diagnosis: Food- and nutrition-related knowledge deficit (DB, LD, HTN, WM)

Sample PES Statement: Food- and nutrition-related knowledge deficit (P) related to lack of exposure to information (E) as evidenced by new diagnosis of diabetes [or prediabetes, lipid disorder, or hypertension] (S).

Sample PES Statement: Food- and nutrition-related knowledge deficit (P) related to sodium content of foods (E) as evidenced by patient requesting assistance with implementing a restricted sodium diet (S).

Nutrition Diagnosis: Not ready for diet/lifestyle change (WM, DB, LD, HTN)

Sample PES Statement: Not ready for lifestyle change (P) related to denial of need to change (precontemplation) (E) as evidenced by reluctance to begin participation in physical activity program (S).

Sample PES Statement: Not ready for lifestyle change (P) related to lack of self-efficacy for making changes (E) as evidenced by patient statements that she cannot lose weight or refrain from salting foods as well as no change in weight or blood pressure level (S).

Nutrition Diagnosis: Limited adherence to nutrition-related recommendations (DB)

Sample PES Statement: Limited adherence to nutrition-related recommendations (P) related to poor understanding or disinterest (E) as evidenced by A1C of 8.5% and food records that indicate patient eats 75 g carbohydrate at breakfast, skips lunch, and eats 150 g carbohydrate at dinner (S).

Nutrition Diagnosis: Physical inactivity (WM, DB, HTN, LD)

Sample PES Statement: Physical inactivity (P) related to perceived lack of time to exercise (E) as evidenced by patient self-reporting less than 30 minutes per week of physical activity (S).

Nutrition Diagnosis: Disordered eating pattern (WM, DB, LD, HTN)

Sample PES Statement: Disordered eating pattern (P) related to restricting foods and eliminating entire food groups to manage weight (E) as evidenced by self-reported food restriction and food rituals surrounding meals and specific foods, as well as low weight for height (S).

Sample PES Statement: Disordered eating pattern (P) related to guilt associated with eating (E) as evidenced by 3 self-induced binging-and-purging episodes per week for 2 consecutive weeks (S).

NUTRITION DIAGNOSIS REFERENCE SHEET

To save time in practice, RDs may want to create their own reference sheet that lists the nutrition diagnoses they use most often and sample PES statements. The following page presents an example of a chart that can be completed and used when needed. For each nutrition diagnosis, take care to use the exact IDNT nutrition diagnosis label and definition and write one or two sample PES statements based on your own patients/clients.

Nutrition Diagnosis	Definition	Etiologies	Signs and Symptoms	Sample PES Statements
1.				
2.				
3.				
4.				

Chapter 4

Nutrition Intervention: The Nutrition Prescription and Disease Management

Nutrition interventions must be integrated into the overall disease management plan. To do this, the RD determines the plan for implementing the nutrition care process—that is, he or she develops a schedule of encounters, establishes measurable and achievable goals, develops the nutrition prescription and MNT priorities, and outlines a plan of action. After the plan of action is determined and prioritized, implementation of nutrition interventions are carried out, monitored and evaluated, and documented.

This chapter provides the EBNPG recommendations that can be used by the RD for determining the nutrition prescription and setting nutrition therapy priorities. Note that nutrition interventions for gestational diabetes and prediabetes and metabolic syndrome are listed at the end of this chapter.

The IDNT nutrition intervention categories that are important for the implementation of the nutrition prescription and MNT for lipid disorders, hypertension, diabetes, and weight management are as follows (2):

- **Nutrition Education**: A formal process to instruct or train patients/clients in a skill or to impart knowledge to help patients/clients voluntarily manage or modify food, nutrition and physical activity

choices and behavior to maintain or improve health (see Chapter 5 for more information on nutrition education).
• **Nutrition Counseling**: a supportive process, characterized by a collaborative counselor–patient/client relationship to establish food, nutrition and physical activity set priorities, goals, and individualized action plans that acknowledge and foster responsibility for self-care to treat an existing condition and promote health. Possible nutrition counseling strategies are summarized in Chapter 5.
• **Coordination of Nutrition Care**: consultation with, referral to, or coordination of nutrition care with other providers, institutions, or agencies that can assist in treating or managing nutrition-related problems.

RELEVANT NUTRITION INTERVENTIONS

In the following sections, recommendations for developing the nutrition prescription are marked with an asterisk. The other recommendations are useful for integrating the nutrition prescription into the overall disease management plan. The EBNPG source and the rating of the recommendation are listed after each recommendation. The EBNPG are identified using this key:

• LD = lipid disorders
• HTN = hypertension
• DB = diabetes
• WM = weight management

Definitions of the ratings are listed on page xv. Other abbreviations are listed on pages xi–xiii.

Lipid Disorders (5)

- A recommended energy intake should be developed and take into consideration whether the goal is weight maintenance or weight loss. Comparison of assessed food and nutrient intake with estimated energy needs can be used to develop strategies to meet the recommendations of the cardioprotective eating pattern. (LD, Consensus)*

- A cardioprotective eating pattern tailored to the individual's needs and providing a fat intake of 25%–35% of kcal is recommended. (LD, Strong)*

- Saturated and *trans* fatty acids (less than 7% of kcal) and less than 200 mg cholesterol per day is recommended. These goals are typically feasible only with fat intake comprising ≤30% of daily calorie intake. (LD, Strong)*

- Calories from saturated and *trans* fatty acids may be replaced by calories from unsaturated fatty acids, complex carbohydrates (fruits, vegetables, and whole grains), and/or protein. For overweight or obese patients, where the goal is reduced energy intake, reduction rather than replacement of calories from saturated fat is warranted. (LD, Strong)*

- Total protein comprising 15% to 20% of energy intake is recommended (vegetable protein is encouraged to help achieve saturated fat and cholesterol goals). (LD, Consensus)*

- Total carbohydrate comprising 45% to 65% of energy intake is recommended (emphasis on high-fiber/complex-carbohydrate sources and avoidance of refined carbohydrate foods). (LD, Consensus)

- For individuals with the metabolic syndrome or elevated TG, a calorie-controlled, cardioprotective food pattern that avoids extremes in carbohydrate and fat intake and includes physical activity is recommended. Non-nutrient-dense calorie sources, including added sugar and alcohol, should be limited as much as possible. Weight loss of 7%–10% of body weight is encouraged if indicated. (LD, Fair)*

- For individuals with elevated TG (≥150 mg/dL), a calorie-controlled, cardioprotective eating pattern that avoids extremes in carbohydrate and fat, and physical activity are recommended. (LD, Fair)*

Hypertension (6)

- The DASH food pattern—which is rich in fruits and vegetables (9–12 servings/d), low-fat dairy (2–3 servings/d), and nuts; low in sodium (less than 2,300 mg/d), total fat, and saturated fat; and adequate in calories for weight management—is recommended. The DASH food pattern reduces SBP by 8–14 mmHg. (HTN, Consensus; LD, Strong)*
- Dietary sodium intake should be limited to 2,300 mg/d. Further reduction in sodium to ≤1,600 mg/d is recommended if treatment goals are not achieved. (HTN, Strong; LD, Strong)*
- To reduce BP, the achievement and maintenance of optimal body weight is recommended. Weight reduction of 22 lb (10 kg) lowers SBP by 5–20 mmHg. (HTN, Strong)*
- Unless contraindicated, at least 30 minutes of moderate-intensity physical activity (eg, brisk walking, swimming laps, bicycling) is recommended for most, if not all, days of the week. Individuals should start slowly and increase activity gradually to achieve goals. Physical activity can reduce SBP by approximately 4–9 mmHg. (LD, Strong; HTN, Consensus)

Diabetes (7,8)

- Macronutrient distribution is based on DRIs for healthy eating. Research does not support any ideal percentage of energy from specific macronutrients for persons with diabetes. (DB, Strong)*

- Cardioprotective nutrition interventions for prevention and treatment of CVD should be implemented in the initial series of encounters. (DB, Strong)*

- A variety of interventions (reduced energy and fat intake, carbohydrate counting, simplified meal plans, healthy food choices, individualized meal planning strategies, exchange lists, insulin-to-carbohydrate ratios, low-fat vegan diets, physical activity, and behavioral strategies) have been shown to improve glycemic control. Any of these interventions may be selected. (DB, Strong)*

- For patients with diabetes, advise that glycemic control is the primary focus of MNT. While decreasing energy intake may improve glycemic control, it is unclear whether weight loss alone will improve glycemic control. (DB, Fair)*

- For people with type 2 diabetes, 90 to 150 minutes of accumulated moderate-intensity aerobic physical activity per week, as well as resistance/strength training three times per week, are recommended. Both aerobic and resistance activities improve glycemic control independent of weight loss, improve insulin sensitivity, and decrease risk of CVD and all-cause mortality. (DB, Strong)

- Individuals with type 1 diabetes are encouraged to engage in regular physical activities. Although exercise is not reported to improve glycemic control in people with type 1 diabetes, such individuals receive the same benefits from exercise as does the general public. (DB, Fair)

- Individuals on insulin or insulin secretagogue therapy should be instructed on the safety guidelines to prevent hypoglycemia (frequent glucose monitoring and possible adjustments in insulin doses or carbohydrate intake). (DB, Fair)

Weight Management (10)

- Goals of weight loss therapy should be individualized with the aim being to reduce body weight at an optimal rate of 1–2 lb per week for the first 6 months and achieve an initial weight loss goal of up to 10% from baseline. (WM, Strong)*
- An individualized reduced calorie diet is the basis of the dietary component of a comprehensive weight management program. Reducing dietary fat and/or carbohydrates is a practical way to create a daily caloric deficit of 500–1,000 kcal below estimated energy needs and can result in a weight loss of 1–2 lb per week for approximately 6 months. (WM, Strong)*
- Total caloric intake should be distributed throughout the day; aim for 4–5 meals and snacks per day, including breakfast. (WM, Fair)*
- Portion control is advised as part of a comprehensive weight management program. (WM, Fair)*
- A comprehensive weight management program includes guidelines for physical activity. The long-term goal is to accumulate at least 30 minutes of moderate intensity physical activity on most, and preferably, all days of the week, unless physical activity is medically contraindicated. (WM, Strong)
- People who have difficulty with self selection and/or portion control may find use of meal replacements (eg, liquid meals, meal bars, and calorie-controlled meals) useful. (WM, Strong)

- Maximum use of multiple strategies for behavior therapy (eg, self monitoring, stress management, stimulus control, problem solving, contingency management, cognitive restructuring, and social support) is recommended. Continued behavioral interventions may be necessary to prevent a return to baseline weight. (WM, Strong)

- The diet component of the weight management program should include individualized nutrition education (eg, reading nutrition labels, recipe modification, and cooking classes). (WM, Fair)

- FDA-approved weight loss medications may be part of a comprehensive weight management program for people who meet the NHLBI criteria for overweight and obesity (see Table 2.8). (WM, Strong)

- RDs should collaborate with other members of the health care team regarding the appropriateness of bariatric surgery for people who meet the NHLBI criteria for obesity. (WM, Strong)

Gestational Diabetes Mellitus (GDM) (9)

- Weight loss during pregnancy is not recommended. In overweight or obese women with GDM, a modest energy restriction (approximately 70% of DRI for pregnant women) is recommended to slow weight gain (GDM, Fair).*

- Based on the DRI, a minimum of 175 g carbohydrate per day is encouraged to provide glucose to the fetal brain and to prevent ketosis. Total carbohydrate should be less than 45% of energy intake to prevent hyperglycemia (GDM, Fair).*

- Protein and fat intake is based on the DRIs for pregnant women (10%–35% and 20%–35% of energy intake, respectively) (GDM, Fair).*

- If usual food intake does not meet DRIs for pregnant women, vitamin and mineral supplementation is encouraged (GDM, Consensus).
- Unless contraindicated, 30 minutes of physical activity per day at least 3 days per week are recommended (GDM, Fair).
- Blood glucose monitoring, including fasting and postprandial levels, is recommended (GDM, Fair).
- Only FDA-approved non-nutritive sweeteners should be consumed during pregnancy. Moderation is encouraged (GDM, Consensus).
- Breastfeeding is encouraged as it results in long-term improvement in the woman's glucose metabolism and may reduce risk of type 2 diabetes in children (GDM, Fair).
- Alcohol consumption, including alcohol used in cooking, is to be avoided (GDM, Consensus).
- Pharmacological therapy (insulin and glyburide) is recommended if optimal blood glucose levels are not maintained with MNT (GDM, Strong).
- Ketone testing is recommended for women who have insufficient energy or carbohydrate intake and those who lose weight (GDM, Fair).
- RDs should monitor and evaluate blood glucose levels, weight change, food intake, physical activity, and pharmacological therapy at each visit (GDM, Strong).
- Weight loss after delivery is advised for women who are overweight or obese and those who gain more weight than is recommended during pregnancy (GDM, Strong).

Prevention of Diabetes and Metabolic Syndrome (15,16,32)

Lifestyle Interventions

- Prevention trials have demonstrated the efficacy of structured programs that emphasize the following lifestyle changes:

○ Moderate weight loss (7% body weight)
○ Regular physical activity (150 min/wk)
○ Reduced intake of calories and dietary fat

Food/Nutrition Interventions*

- For good health, encourage a food pattern that includes carbohydrate from fruits, vegetables, whole grain and high-fiber foods, legumes and nuts, and low-fat or fat-free milk.
- Limit saturated fat and *trans* fatty acids to less than 7% of total energy intake and food cholesterol to less than 200 mg/d. Choose unsaturated fats from vegetables, fish, nuts, and legumes.
- Recommend two or more servings of fish per week (with the exception of commercially fried fish filets) for n-3 polyunsaturated fatty acids.
- Limit sodium intake to 2,300 mg/d by choosing foods low in sodium and limiting the amount of salt added to food.
- Minimize intake of beverages and foods with added sugars.
- Adults who choose to drink alcohol should limit alcohol intake. The limit for men is two drinks per day. The limit for women is one drink per day.

Physical Activity Recommendations

- For fitness, adults should aim for 30 minutes of moderate physical activity (eg, walking 3–4 mph) in addition to usual activity, on most days of the week.
- For prevention of weight gain, adults should aim for 60 minutes of moderate-to-vigorous activity (to increase energy expenditure by 150–200 kcal/d) on most days of the week while not exceeding energy intake requirements.

- To avoid regain of weight loss, adults should aim for 60–90 minutes of moderate-intensity physical activity per day (250–300 min/wk or approximately 2,000 kcal/wk) while not exceeding energy intake requirements.
- Vigorous-intensity physical activities and being active for longer durations will provide greater benefits, such as for maintenance of weight or achievement of weight control goals.
- Cardiovascular conditioning, stretching exercises for flexibility, and resistance training for muscle strength are also recommended.

Medication Recommendations

- For patients at high risk of diabetes or metabolic syndrome, pharmacologic treatment may be considered. (However, the FDA has not approved any drugs to prevent diabetes.)
- Metformin and acarbose are safe and have been shown to decrease the development of diabetes from prediabetes.
- Thiazolidinediones also reduce the risk for progression from prediabetes to diabetes. However, there are safety concerns with thiazolidinediones, including congestive heart failure or fractures.
- For diabetes prevention, the American Diabetes Association recommends that only metformin be considered. Issues of cost, adverse effects, and lack of persistence of effect are related to other drugs (15).
- In addition to lifestyle modifications, medications for hypertension and dyslipidemia may be required.

Chapter 5

Nutrition Intervention: Nutrition Education and Nutrition Counseling

NUTRITION EDUCATION

To implement nutrition interventions and self-management, patients/clients need knowledge and skills. Nutrition education begins in a series of initial encounters with the RD, which are ideally followed by ongoing nutrition education and counseling. Initial encounters often focus on nutrition education in basic food, eating, and physical activity skills that have been prioritized by the RD and the individual client/patient. In-depth information and additional skills and topics may be added as nutrition education progresses. The possible topics are numerous and vary according to the individual's characteristics, needs, and desires. Outcomes must be identified and the effectiveness of nutrition interventions continually evaluated.

To help RDs identify potential nutrition education topics, the following sections outline specific MNT recommendations related to food and nutrients from the EBNPG. The EBNPG are identified after each recommendation using this key:

- **LD** = lipid disorders
- **HTN** = hypertension

- **DB** = diabetes
- **WM** = weight management

Definitions of the ratings that follow each recommendation are listed on page xv. Other abbreviations are listed on pages xi–xiii.

MACRONUTRIENTS

Fat Components and Cardioprotective Nutrition Therapy

- Cardioprotective nutrition interventions for the prevention and treatment of CVD include reduction in saturated and *trans* fatty acids and dietary cholesterol as well as interventions to improve blood pressure. (LD, Strong; DB, Strong)
- Intake of saturated and *trans* fatty acids should be as limited as possible and less than 7% of total energy intake. (LD, Strong)
- Saturated fatty acids may be replaced by mono-unsaturated or polyunsaturated fats, complex carbohydrates, and/or protein. (LD, Strong)
- n-3 fatty acids, preferably from fish, are recommended. For individuals without CHD, two fish servings (4 oz each) per week are recommended. For individuals with CHD, two or more fish servings per week are recommended. (LD, Fair)
- Foods rich in plant-derived n-3 fatty acids can be recommended to reduce the risk of CVD. (LD, Fair)
- If the individual does not eat food sources of n-3 fatty acids, 1 g of EPA and DHA n-3 supplements may be advised for secondary prevention. n-3 fatty acids do not seem to lower BP. Consumption of more than 3 g of n-3 fatty acids per day may cause gastrointestinal symptoms. (LD, Fair; HTN, Fair)

- If an individual has elevated TG (>200 mg/dL), then in addition to lifestyle therapies, high-dose supplemental EPA/DHA (2 to 4 g/d) may be used under medical supervision. (LD, Strong)

Carbohydrate

Carbohydrate and Diabetes

- For individuals on MNT alone, glucose-lowering medications, or fixed insulin doses, it is recommended that meal and snack carbohydrate intake be consistent from day to day. (DB, Strong)
- For individuals with type 1 or type 2 diabetes who adjust their mealtime insulin doses or are on insulin pump therapy, it is recommended that insulin doses be adjusted to match carbohydrate intake (insulin-to-carbohydrate ratios). (DB, Strong)

Carbohydrate and Weight Management

- During the first 6 months of weight loss intervention, low-carbohydrate diets are associated with a greater weight loss than reduced-calorie or reduced-fat diets, but these differences are not clinically or statistically significant after 1 year. (WM, Fair)

Sucrose

- If people with diabetes choose to eat foods containing sucrose, the sucrose-containing foods can be substituted for other carbohydrate foods in the meal plan. (DB, Strong)

Fiber

- A cardioprotective diet should include 25–30 g fiber from food per day, with special emphasis on soluble fiber (7–13 g/d). Foods rich in soluble fiber include fruits, vegetables, whole grains (especially high-fiber cereals, oatmeal) and legumes (especially beans). Diets high in total and soluble fiber, as part of a cardio-protective eating patttern, can reduce TC by 2%–3% and LDL-C by up to 7%. (LD, Strong; DB, Strong)

- Consumption of soluble fiber may or may not help reduce BP. (HTN, Weak)
- In research studies, intake of 44–50 g fiber per day improved glycemia. However, more usual fiber intakes (up to 25 g/d) have not demonstrated beneficial effects on glycemia. (DB, Strong)

Non-nutritive Sweeteners

- If individuals choose to consume products containing FDA-approved non-nutritive sweeteners at levels that do not exceed the ADIs, they should be aware that some of these products contain energy and carbohydrate from other sources that need to be accounted for (DB, Fair)

Glycemic Index

- Research on the efficacy of the glycemic index as a method of meal planning is inconclusive. Studies comparing high– vs low–glycemic index diets report mixed effects on A1C and lipids. (DB, Fair)
- A low–glycemic index diet is *not* recommended for weight loss or weight maintenance as it has not been shown to be effective. (WM, Strong)

Protein

- Consumption of protein may or may not help reduce BP. (HTN, Weak)
- Individuals with type 1 or type 2 diabetes and normal renal function do not need to change their usual intake

of protein (approximately 15%–20% of daily energy intake). Although protein has an acute effect on insulin secretion, usual protein intake has minimal effects on glucose, lipids, or insulin concentrations. (DB, Fair)

• In individuals with diabetic nephropathy, the recommended protein intake is less than 1 g per kilogram of body weight per day. (DB, Fair)

• In individuals with late-stage diabetic nephropathy (CKD Stages 3–5), monitoring of hypoalbuminemia (an indicator of malnutrition) and energy intake is recommended. Changes in protein and energy intake should be made to correct deficits. (DB, Fair)

SPECIFIC FOODS

Fruits and Vegetables

• Advise consumption of 5 to 10 servings of fruits and vegetables per day, based on research reporting reductions in BP after the consumption of the DASH food pattern or a diet rich in fruits and vegetables. (HTN, Strong)

Plant Stanols and Sterols

• Daily intake of foods containing plant sterol and stanol ester-enriched foods consumed 2 to 3 times per day for a total consumption of 2-3 g/d can reduce TC by 4%–11% and LDL-C by 7%–15%. For maximal effectiveness, enriched foods should be eaten with other foods. (LD, Strong)

Soy Foods

• Consuming 25–50 g soy protein per day in place of animal protein can reduce TC by 0%–20% and LDL-C by 4%–24%. (LD, Fair)

• Consumption of soy foods may or may not help reduce BP. (HTN, Weak)

Nuts

• Consumption of 5 ounces (~900 kcal) of nuts (walnuts, almonds, peanuts, macadamia, pistachios, or pecans) per week is associated with reduced CHD risk. Nuts should be isocalorically incorporated into a cardioprotective eating pattern. (LD, Fair)

Dairy Foods

• To meet current nutritional recommendations, the diet of a comprehensive weight management program should include 3–4 servings of low-fat dairy foods per day. (WM, Fair)

Garlic

• Consumption of garlic may or may not help reduce BP. (HTN, Weak)

Cocoa and Chocolate

• Cocoa or chocolate may or may not help reduce BP. (HTN, Weak)

Caffeine

• Suggest BP monitoring to individuals who consume caffeine. Although acute intake of caffeine increases BP, the effect of chronic caffeine intake on BP is unclear. (HTN, Weak)

Alcohol

• A maximum of one drink per day for women and up to two drinks per day for men is associated with reduced CVD risk. There is no evidence that one type of alcohol is better than another for risk reduction. Evidence does not justify recommending that non-drinkers begin drinking alcohol, and alcohol should not be consumed when contraindicated. (LD, Fair; HTN, Consensus)

- A reduction in alcohol consumption to a maximum of one drink per day for women and two drinks per day for men may reduce SBP by approximately 2–4 mmHg. (HTN, Consensus)

MICRONUTRIENTS

Sodium

- Daily sodium intake should be limited to no more than 2,300 mg (100 mmol). Reduction of sodium to the recommended level can lower SBP by approximately 2–8 mmHg. (HTN, Strong)
- If BP treatment goals are not achieved by limiting sodium to 2,300 mg/d, the DASH food pattern and/or reduction of sodium intake to 1,600 mg/d are recommended. (HTN, Strong)

Potassium

- To reduce BP, consumption of adequate food sources of potassium is recommended. (HTN, Fair)

Magnesium

- The effect of magnesium as a single nutrient on BP is unknown. (HTN, Fair)

Calcium

- The effect of calcium as a single nutrient on BP is unclear. (HTN, Fair)

Antioxidants and Vitamins

- Antioxidant-rich foods such as fruits, vegetables, whole grains, and nuts are associated with reduced CVD. (LD, Consensus)
- Vitamin E, vitamin C, and beta-carotene supplements should *not* be recommended to reduce CVD risk. Research indicates that high doses of antioxidants (above the RDA) do not provide cardiovascular benefit and may cause harm or even shorten life. (LD, Strong)
- Supplemental vitamin E, vitamin C, beta-carotene, and selenium should not be taken with simvastatin–niacin drug combinations. Supplemental beta-carotene also cannot be recommended for individuals who smoke. Research indicates that in these situations there is increased CVD risk with supplement use. (LD, Fair)
- Consumption of vitamin C or vitamin E may or may not be beneficial for the reduction of BP. (The effect of increased vitamin C or vitamin E intake on blood pressure is unclear.) (HTN, Weak)
- Food intake should be planned to meet the DRIs for folate, vitamin B-6, and vitamin B-12. Although supplemental B vitamins may lower homocysteine in people with high homocysteine levels (>13 mcmol/L), this has not reduced CVD risk and may be harmful. (LD, Strong)
- Supplemental doses of folate, vitamin B-6, and vitamin B-12 should not be recommended; they are not be beneficial for the prevention of CHD. (LD, Weak)

Coenzyme Q_{10}

- Evidence is lacking for an association between coenzyme Q_{10} and CHD. The clinical significance of normalizing CoQ10 levels in people treated with statin medications is inconclusive. (LD, Weak)

NUTRITION COUNSELING

The combined use of behavior theory and cognitive behavioral theory has a greater impact than any individual theory or technique used alone in facilitating modification of targeted food habits, weight, and cardiovascular and diabetes risk factors (40,41). However, the incorporation of a variety of techniques in one session with a client/patient may seem complex and challenging. The following "five A's" describe steps that can guide the RD in starting an education/counseling session and implementing the best of several behavioral change strategies for each part of the session (42):

- Step 1: Ask
- Step 2: Assess
- Step 3: Advise
- Step 4: Agree
- Step 5: Arrange

Taken together, these five A's provide a workable framework that can integrate other counseling models.

Step 1: Ask

The "ask" step emphasizes the importance of questions as the RD aims to develop a relationship with the client. The following tactics are essential to this step:

- Use motivational interviewing techniques (Table 5.1) throughout the nutrition education/counseling session (43,44).
- Establish rapport by demonstrating the ability to be open, genuine, caring, and empathetic.

Table 5.1   Motivational Interviewing Techniques

Ask open-ended questions:
- Encourage clients to do the talking.
- Do not ask questions that elicit a "yes" or "no" response.

Express empathy:
- Acknowledge the client's difficulties.
- Validate the client's thoughts and feelings.

Listen reflectively:
- Rephrase the client's responses to reflect what you think you heard.
- State back what you think the client meant.

Support self-efficacy:
- Provide choices and reassure the client about expected outcomes.

Express sympathy:
- Express acceptance and understanding.
- Use reflective listening and expect ambivalence.

Explore discrepancies:
- Let individuals explore their reasons for changing or not changing behaviors.

Roll with resistance:
- Avoid arguments.
- Avoid judging and labeling.
- Change strategies if individuals show resistance.

Summarize:
- Rephrase the overall content and meaning of the conversation.
- Reveal any ambiguity.

Promote empowerment:
- Recognize that individuals are source of their own solutions, and each individual is in charge of and responsible for his or her own care.

Source: Adapted with permission from reference 43: VanWormer JJ, Boucher JL. Motivational interviewing and diabetes education: fostering commitment to change. *On the Cutting Edge: Diabetes Care and Education.* 2003;24(4):14–16.

• Begin each session by asking questions to determine what the client wants to know and accomplish and what you can do to be of assistance.

Step 2: Assess

In the "assess" step, the RD evaluates the client's readiness to change (Table 5.2) (45,46) as part of the nutrition

Table 5.2   Transtheoretical Model of Intentional Behavior Change (Stages of Change)

Precontemplation
- Attitude toward lifestyle change is "Never":
  - Individuals in this stage have no intention of changing behavior in foreseeable future.
  - They are unaware they have a problem and resistant to efforts to modify behavior.
- Suggested interventions for health professionals:
  - Personalize risk factors.
  - Discuss health concern and its implications.

Contemplation
- Attitude toward lifestyle change is "Someday":
  - Individuals in this stage are aware they have a problem and seriously thinking about change.
  - They have not yet made a commitment to take action in the near future.
- Suggested interventions for health professionals:
  - Provide basic information.
  - Help the client see that the pros of change outweigh the cons.

Preparation
- Attitude toward lifestyle change is "Soon":
  - Individuals are in the stage of decision making.
  - They will commit to take action within the next 30 days.
  - They begin making small behavioral changes.
- Suggested interventions for health professionals:
  - Set a date to start.
  - Teach specific "how-to" skills.

(continues on next page)

Table 5.2   Transtheoretical Model of Intentional Behavior Change (Stages of Change) (continued)

Action
- Attitude toward lifestyle change is "Now":
  - Individuals are making notable overt efforts to change.
  - They target behaviors that can be modified to an acceptable criterion.
  - They may not consistently carry out new behaviors.
- Suggested interventions for health professionals:
  - Implement counseling strategies.
  - Continue to reinforce and support their decision to change.
  - Discuss the difference between a lapse vs relapse.

Maintenance
- Attitude toward lifestyle change is "Forever":
  - Individuals are working to stabilize behavior change and to avoid relapse.
  - They sustain their behavior change for at least 6 months.
- Suggested interventions for health professionals:
  - Provide support; encourage behavior maintenance strategies.
  - Continue relapse prevention counseling.

Source: Data are from references 45 and 46.

assessment (see Chapter 1 for more information on nutrition assessment).

When using Stages of Change, the RD's objective is to help the client to achieve the action or maintenance stage for the desired health behavior:

- If clients are in the **precontemplation** stage, the goal is to help them recognize they are at risk for a health problem.
- If clients are in the **contemplation** stage, aim to help them believe their risk of disease is serious and that personal actions make a difference. The benefits must outweigh the barriers to get clients to the next step.

- If clients are in the **preparation** stage, provide encouragement and set a start date.
- If clients are in the **action** stage, help them implement the strategies that individuals who have made lifestyle changes identify as the most helpful (Table 5.3) (41,47). Use tools such as the following:
  - Food and activity records so client becomes aware of changes he/she needs and is willing to make (also helpful in the preparation stage)
  - Goal setting so client determines to make realistic changes
- If clients are in the **maintenance** stage, provide support and continue encouragement to facilitate behaviors that maintain the healthful change (Table 5.4) (41,47).

Table 5.3   Strategies for Modifying Behavior

Self-monitoring

- Record your target behaviors and factors associated with your behaviors to increase awareness of how you behave; participants report this strategy to be most helpful.
- Record the "what, where, and when" of eating and physical activity (individuals with diabetes should also keep blood glucose monitoring records).

Goal setting

- To achieve incremental improvements, set specific short-term targets for your behavior habits.

Stimulus control

- Identify triggers associated with your problem behaviors; design strategies to break links.
- Restrict environmental factors associated with inappropriate behaviors.
- Eat at specific times; set aside time and place for physical activities.
- Avoid purchasing foods that you find difficult to eat in moderation.

(continues on next page)

Table 5.3   Strategies for Modifying Behavior (continued)

Cognitive restructuring

- Change perceptions, thoughts, or beliefs that undermine your behavior-change efforts.
- Change thinking patterns from unrealistic goals to realistic and achievable goals.
- Move thinking patterns away from self-rejection and toward self-acceptance.

Contingency management

- Use rewards (tangible or verbal) to improve performance of specific behaviors or recognize when specified goals are reached (participants rated this strategy as least helpful).
- Create contracts to formalize agreements; contracts should be short term and focus on increasing healthful behaviors.

Stress management

- Stress is a primary predictor of relapse; therefore, methods to reduce stress and tension are critical.
- Try tension reduction skills such as diaphragmatic breathing, progressive muscle relaxation, and/or meditation.
- Regular physical activity helps reduce stress.

Source: Adapted with permission from reference 47: Klein S, Burke LE, Gray GA, Glair S, Allison DB, Pi-Sunyer X, Hong Y, Eckel RH. Clinical implications of obesity with specific focus on cardiovascular disease. A statement for professionals from the American Heart Association Council on Nutrition, Physical Activity, and Metabolism. *Circulation.* 2004;110:2952–2967.

Step 3: Advise

The "advise" step uses a client-centered framework:

- Focus on the concerns of the client/patient.
- Allow client to be the expert of him or herself.
- Adapt nutrition interventions to meet the client's needs, wants, priorities, preferences and expectations. (See Chapter 4 for more information on nutrition interventions.)

Table 5.4   Strategies for Maintaining Behavior Change

Structured programs with ongoing contact
- Individuals aiming to achieve and maintain goals require assistance from structured programs with consistent follow-up contacts.
- Maintain visits, telephone calls, or Internet communication to promote adherence with recommended lifestyle changes.

Social support
- Use social support—family, peer support, self-help or worksite groups or involvement in social activities—to maintain successful behavior change.

Physical activity and exercise
- Promote regular involvement in physical activities—individuals who exercise regularly are also more likely to maintain other health behaviors.

Relapse prevention
- Recognize that lapses in behavior can be anticipated in certain situations (eg, travel, social situations, celebrations, stressful situations, loneliness) and develop skills for these situations.
- Individuals can practice coping strategies to handle high-risk situations (eg, stress management, social situation skills).

Source: Adapted with permission from reference 47: Klein S, Burke LE, Gray GA, Glair S, Allison DB, Pi-Sunyer X, Hong Y, Eckel RH. Clinical implications of obesity with specific focus on cardiovascular disease. A statement for professionals from the American Heart Association Council on Nutrition, Physical Activity, and Metabolism. *Circulation.* 2004;110:2952–2967.

Step 4: Agree

In the "agree" step, the RD facilitates the client's process of setting his or her own short-term goals related to nutrition, physical activity, or glucose monitoring (if appropriate) and helps outline the client's potential methods for accomplishing lifestyle change.

Scaling questions are recommended. For example:

- "On a scale of zero to 10, with zero being not important and 10 being very important, how important is it for you to modify XX behavior?" can be used to evaluate a client's goals.

• "On a scale of zero to 10, with zero being not important and 10 being very important, how confident are you that you can XX?" can be used to evaluate a client's plans.

Step 5: Arrange

In the "arrange" step, the RD helps implement a plan for follow-up adapted to the client's goals and needs, the client's level of support from family and friends, and available resources. Crucial tasks include the following:

• Schedule follow-up visits.
• Provide contact information for future questions.
• Make referrals and/or provide contact information for other providers.

Chapter 6

Nutrition Monitoring and Evaluation and Documentation

NUTRITION MONITORING AND EVALUATION

The purpose of nutrition monitoring and evaluation is to evaluate the progress made by the client/patient and determine whether goals are being met. If the client has made all the lifestyle changes he or she can or is willing to make and medical goals have not been achieved, the RD must notify the referral source so changes in medical therapy, such as added or adjusted medications, can be made.

The following are nutrition care outcomes that may be used for monitoring and evaluation of MNT provided for lipid disorders, hypertension, diabetes, and weight management (2):

- Changes in nutrition-related physical signs and symptoms associated with anthropometric, biochemical, and physical examination parameters
- Nutrition-related behavioral and environmental outcomes, such as changes in nutrition-related knowledge, behaviors, access, or ability that may impact food and nutrient intake
- Food and nutrient intake outcomes
- Nutrition-related patient/client-centered outcomes associated with a patient/client's perception of his or her nutrition intervention and its impact on his or her life

To effectively monitor outcomes, it is essential that RDs know expected outcomes from MNT interventions and when to evaluate them (see Table 6.1). However, it is important to note that the expected outcomes are averages—some clients will exceed the expected outcomes whereas others may not achieve a positive outcome.

Table 6.1   Effectiveness of Medical Nutrition Therapy

Endpoint and Expected Outcomes	When to Evaluate
Lipids • TC: 24–32 mg/dL (10%–13%) decrease • LDL-C: 18–25 mg/dL (12%–16%) decrease • TG: 15–17 mg/dL (8%) decrease • HDL-C: 3 mg/dL (7%) decrease with no exercise; no decrease in HDL-C with exercise.	6 weeks after start of MNT; if goals are not achieved, intensify MNT and evaluate again in 6 weeks.
Blood pressure: • Individual with HTN, not on medication: 14 mmHg decrease SBP; 7 mmHg decrease DBP • Nonhypertensive individuals: 9 mmHg decrease SBP; 6 mmHg decrease in DBP	At every medical visit.
Glycemic control: • A1C: 1%–2% decrease (15%–22% improvement) • Fasting plasma glucose: 50 mg/dL decrease	6 weeks to 3 months after start of MNT.
Weight: • 5–8.5 kg (5%–10%) decrease during the first 6 months of therapy • Maintenance to 12 months • 3–6 kg (3%–6%) at 4 years	At every encounter.

Source: Data are from references 22, 24, 30, and 48.

NUTRITION MONITORING AND EVALUATION RECOMMENDATIONS

The following sections outline specific nutrition monitoring and evaluation recommendations from the EBNPG. The EBNPG are identified after each recommendation using this key:

- **LD** = lipid disorders
- **HTN** = hypertension
- **DB** = diabetes
- **WM** = weight management

Definitions of the ratings that follow each recommendation are listed on page xv. Other abbreviations are listed on pages xi–xiii.

Disorders of Lipid Metabolism

- Monitor and evaluate at each visit: food, beverage, and nutrient intake (energy intake; serving sizes; meal/snack pattern; fat intake; types of fat; cholesterol, carbohydrate, fiber, and micronutrient intake; bioactive substances [alcohol intake, plant stanols and sterols, soy protein, psyllium, fish oil]) and compare to desired individual outcomes related to the nutrition diagnosis and intervention. (LD, Consensus)
- Monitor and evaluate medication (see Table 2.9 for lipid treatment guidelines) and herbal supplements: use, knowledge, food and nutrient administration (individual's experience with food), behavior, factors affecting access to food, and physical activity and function. (LD, Consensus)
- Monitor and evaluate anthropometric data (BMI, waist circumference or waist-to-hip ratio) and compare to desired outcomes related to the nutrition diagnosis and intervention. (LD, Strong)

- Monitor and evaluate biochemical data, medical tests, and procedures (lipid profile, blood pressure, fasting glucose, and other values as appropriate) and compare with desired individual outcomes related to the nutrition diagnosis and intervention. (LD, Consensus)
- Monitor and evaluate energy and macronutrient needs, revise goals as appropriate, and develop strategies to meet the recommendations of the cardioprotective eating pattern. Determine what future action is warranted. (LD, Consensus)

Blood Pressure

- Monitor and evaluate the effectiveness of therapy by blood pressure measurement. (HTN, Consensus)
- A treatment goal of <140/90 mmHg is recommended for individuals without comorbidities. (HTN, Consensus)
- For individuals with hypertension and diabetes or renal disease, a treatment goal of <130/80 mmHg is recommended. (HTN, Consensus)

Glucose Monitoring

- For individuals on nutrition therapy alone or nutrition therapy in combination with glucose-lowering medications, self-monitoring of blood glucose (SMBG) is recommended. Frequency and timing are dependent on diabetes management goals and therapies (ie, MNT, diabetes medications, and physical activity). (DB, Fair)
- For persons with type 1 or type 2 diabetes on insulin therapy, at least three to eight blood glucose tests per day are recommended to determine the adequacy of the insulin dose(s) and guide adjustments in insulin dose(s), food intake, and physical activity. Some insulin regimens require more frequent testing

to establish the best integrated therapy (insulin, food, and activity). Once established, some insulin regimens will require less frequent SMBG. (See Appendix B for insulin strategies.) (DB, Strong)

- Persons with unexplained elevations in A1C or unexplained hypoglycemia and hyperglycemia may benefit from continuous glucose monitoring (CGM) or more frequent SMBG. It is essential that persons with diabetes receive education on how to calibrate CGM and interpret CGM results. (DB, Fair)
- Monitor and evaluate food intake, medication, metabolic control (glycemia, lipids, and BP) and anthropometric measurements and physical activity. (DB, Strong)
- Blood glucose (BG) results are primarily used in evaluating the achievement of goals and effectiveness of MNT. Glucose monitoring results can be used to determine whether adjustments in foods and meals will be sufficient to achieve BG goals or if medication additions or adjustments need to be combined with MNT. (DB, Consensus)

Weight Management

- Body weight and waist circumference are used to determine the effectiveness of therapy in the reassessment. (WM, Fair)
- Individualized weight loss therapy goals are to reduce body weight at an optimal rate of 1 to 2 lb/week for the first 6 months and achieve an initial weight loss goal of up to 10% from baseline. (WM, Strong)

DOCUMENTATION OF NUTRITION CARE

Documentation in the patient/client's medical record serves as a communication tool for members of the health

Table 6.2 Key NCP-Related Charting Elements for Medical Records

Nutrition assessment
- Date and time of assessment.
- Pertinent data collected and comparisons with standards (eg, food and nutrition history, biochemical data, anthropometric measurements, client history, and medical therapy and supplement use).
- Patient/client's readiness to learn, food and nutrition-related knowledge, and potential for change.
- Physical activity history and goals.
- Reason for discontinuation of nutrition therapy, if appropriate.

Nutrition diagnosis
- Date and time.
- Concise written statement of nutrition diagnosis (or nutrition diagnoses) written in the PES format (problem, etiology, signs and symptoms). If there is no existing or predicted nutrition problem that requires a nutrition intervention, state "no nutrition diagnosis at this time."

Nutrition intervention
- Date and time.
- Specific treatment goals and expected outcomes.
- Recommended nutrition prescription and nutrition interventions (individualized for the patient).
- Any adjustments to plan and justifications.
- Patient/client's attitude regarding recommendations.
- Changes in patient/client's level of understanding and food-related behaviors (these must be documented along with changes in clinical or functional outcomes).
- Referrals made and resources used.
- Any other information relevant to providing care and monitoring progress over time.
- Plans for follow-up and frequency of care.

Nutrition monitoring and evaluation
- Date and time.
- Specific nutrition outcome indicators and results relevant to the nutrition diagnosis (or diagnoses) and intervention plans and goals, compared with previous status or reference goals.
- Progress toward nutrition intervention goals.
- Factors facilitating or hindering progress.
- Other positive or negative outcomes.
- Future plans for nutrition care, monitoring, and follow-up or discharge.

Source: Data are from reference 49.

care team. Concise, timely, accurate, and high-quality information provides evidence that the individualized nutrition care plan developed by the RD is effective. The medical record also serves as a legal document of what was done and not done and supports reimbursement of nutrition services billed to insurance carriers. Furthermore, accrediting organizations review charts to ensure that nutrition services are provided in a timely and effective manner using an interdisciplinary approach. Such chart reviews support their decisions in the certification process.

There are many different formats available for medical record documentation. The appropriate format depends on where the RD practices, and whether electronic health records are used. Regardless of the specific format, the RD can document using the steps of the Nutrition Care Process (eg, A = Nutrition Assessment, D = Nutrition Diagnosis, I = Nutrition Intervention, ME = Nutrition Monitoring and Evaluation). RDs who use electronic health records can incorporate the IDNT standardized language into the electronic health record to facilitate database queries and data compilation. Table 6.2 lists key charting elements to consider when documenting each NCP step (49).

Appendix A

Useful Formulas

CALORIE-RELATED FORMULAS

Body Fat–Calorie Relationship

1 lb body fat = 3,500 kcal

Calorie Content

1 g carbohydrate = 4 kcal
1 g protein = 4 kcal
1 g fat = 9 kcal
1 g alcohol = 7 kcal

CONVERSIONS

Système International (SI) Units and Conventional Units

Glucose	_____ mmol/L × 18	=	_____ mg/dL
Glucose:	_____ mg/dL × 0.0555	=	_____ mmol/L
Cholesterol:	_____ mmol/L × 38.7	=	_____ mg/dL
Cholesterol:	_____ mg/dL × 0.02586	=	_____ mmol/L
Triglycerides:	_____ mmol/L × 88.6	=	_____ mg/dL
Triglycerides:	_____ mg/dL × 0.0112	=	_____ mmol/L
Insulin:	_____ mmol/L ÷ 6.0	=	_____ mcU/mL
C-peptide:	_____ mmol/L × 3.03	=	_____ ng/mL
Sodium:	_____ mmol × 23	=	_____ mg
Sodium chloride:	_____ mmol × 58 (23 + 35)	=	_____ mg
Potassium:	_____ mmol × 39	=	_____ mg
Calcium:	_____ mmol × 40	=	_____ mg
Vitamin D (25[OH]D):	_____ ng/mL × 2.496	=	_____ nmol/L
Vitamin D (25[OH]D):	_____ nmol/L × 0.4	=	_____ ng/mL

Conventional-Metric Conversions

1 inch	=	2.54 cm
1 lb	=	0.4536 kg
1 oz	=	28.35 g
1 fl oz	=	29.57 mL
1 g	=	0.0353 oz
1 g	=	0.0022 lb
1 kg	=	2.21 lb

OTHER COMMONLY USED FORMULAS

Body Mass Index

$$\text{BMI} = \text{Weight (kg)}/\text{Height (m)}^2$$

$$\text{BMI} = [\text{Weight (lb)}/\text{Height (in)}^2] \times 703$$

Mifflin-St Jeor Equation for Estimated Resting Metabolic Rate

When indirect calorimetry is not possible, the Mifflin-St Jeor equation is recommended for estimating RMR in overweight and obese individuals. Use actual weight to derive the most accurate estimate (50).

$$\text{Men: RMR} = (10 \times \text{Weight}) + (6.25 \times \text{Height}) - (5 \times \text{Age}) + 5$$

$$\text{Women: RMR} = (10 \times \text{Weight}) + (6.25 \times \text{Height}) - (5 \times \text{Age}) - 161$$

Where: Weight is measured in kg; height in cm; age in years.

Non-HDL Cholesterol

$$\text{Non-HDL-C} = \text{TC} - \text{HDL-C}$$

Teaching Tips for Diabetes

HYPOGLYCEMIA

Signs and Symptoms

- **Mild hypoglycemia**: sweating, trembling, difficulty concentrating, lightheadedness, lack of coordination
- **Severe hypoglycemia**: inability to self-treat due to mental confusion, lethargy, or unconsciousness

Treatment

- Immediate treatment with carbohydrate is essential.
- If blood glucose is less than 70 mg/dL:
  - Treat with 15 g carbohydrate, preferably in the form of glucose products.
  - Wait 15 minutes then retest blood glucose; if it remains less than 70 mg/dL, treat with another 15 g carbohydrate.
  - Repeat testing and treating until blood glucose returns to normal range.
  - If there is more than 1 hour until next meal, retest blood glucose and add an additional 15 g carbohydrate to maintain blood glucose in normal range.
- Severe hypoglycemia needs to be treated by someone knowledgeable about diabetes. If the patient cannot swallow well, glucagon must be used instead of oral treatment.

SICK DAY GUIDELINES FOR
PERSONS WITH DIABETES

- Take usual doses of insulin even if you are vomiting and unable to eat. Due to the stress of illness, supplemental insulin doses may be needed.
- Take usual doses of glucose-lowering medications.
- Check blood glucose levels and urine (or blood) for ketones every 2 to 4 hours. Test for ketones if blood glucose level is greater than 250 mg/dL
- Call your health care team if premeal blood glucose remains greater than 250 mg/dL and/or when ketones are moderate or large.
- Drink 8 oz liquids every hour or small quantities every 15 to 30 minutes.
- Eat about 15 g carbohydrate every 1 to 2 hours or 45–50 g every 3 to 4 hours (choices include regular soft drinks, soup, juices, gelatin desserts, or ice cream).
- Seek medical attention if you have:
  ○ Temperature greater than 100 degrees Fahrenheit
  ○ Blood glucose levels that are difficult to control, with or without ketones
  ○ Vomiting and are unable to take fluids for more than 4 hours
  ○ Persistent diarrhea
  ○ Severe abdominal pain, difficulty breathing, or confusion
  ○ Other unexplained symptoms
  ○ Illness that persists more than 24 hours

PHYSICAL ACTIVITY GUIDELINES
FOR INSULIN USERS

- Measure blood glucose levels before, during, and after physical activity.
- For unplanned activity, eat extra carbohydrate (15–30 g per 30 minutes of exercise) before exercise. Insulin dose may need to be decreased after exercise.
- If you take rapid-acting insulin and plan to exercise within 3 hours of meal-related insulin dose, decrease rapid-acting insulin.
- Patients on insulin pumps may suspend or decrease their basal rate during and after exercise.
- During long–duration exercise, you may need to eat carbohydrate.
- After exercise, you may need to eat extra carbohydrate or decrease your insulin dose.

USEFUL INSULIN STRATEGIES

Table B.1   Insulin Strategies for Type 1 Diabetes

Physiological insulin regimens or insulin pumps:
- Average insulin dose: 0.4 to 1.0 units/kg/d with higher amounts during puberty.
- 50% basal (background) and 50% bolus (mealtime, divided between meals) insulins.
- Insulin-to-carbohydrate ratios can vary between 1 unit insulin per 5 g carbohydrate and 1 unit insulin per 25 g carbohydrate.
- Correction bolus algorithms based on insulin sensitivity or correction factor (CF):
  - CF is the estimated number of mg/dL the BG will decrease during a 2- to 4-hour period from injection of 1 unit rapid-acting insulin.
  - Using the "1700 rule," CF = 1700 ÷ Total daily insulin dose.

Source: Data are from reference 39.

Table B.2   Insulin Strategies for Type 2 Diabetes

Initial Insulin Regimen	*Nutrition Guidelines*
Basal insulin added to glucose-lowering medications: 1 dose (often given at bedtime)	• 3 meals/d (women: 2–4 carbohydrate choices/meal; men: 3–5 carbohydrate choices/meal). • Snacks are not needed.
Premixed insulin: 2 doses (1 each before breakfast and evening meal)	• 3 meals at consistent times with consistent carbohydrate intake. • Individuals on NPH and/or regular insulin may need small snacks.
Basal and bolus insulin: background and mealtime insulin doses	• Initially, a consistent carbohydrate intake. • Initiate insulin-to-carbohydrate ratio when patient is ready.

Source: Data are from reference 51.

Appendix C

Professional Resources

GENERAL FOOD AND NUTRITION RESOURCES

Academy of Nutrition and Dietetics:
- Web site: www.eatright.org
- Evidence Analysis Library:
  www.andevidencelibrary.com
- Evidence-based publications and toolkits:
  www.andevidencelibrary.com/store
- Nutrition Care Process: www.eatright.org/
  HealthProfessionals/content.aspx?id=7077
- Nutrition Care Manual:
  www.nutritioncaremanual.org
  (preview site: www.adancm.com/demo)
- Position papers: www.eatright.org/positions
- RDs Weigh In (blog): www.eatright.org/media/
  blog.aspx?blogid=269
- Vegetarian Nutrition Practice Group:
  www.vegetariannutrition.net

Collage Video's Guide to Exercise Videos:
  www.CollageVideo.com
Dietary Reference Intakes: www.fnic.nal.usda.gov
Institute of Medicine: www.iom.edu
Intuitive Eating: www.intuitiveeating.com
MedlinePlus: www.medlineplus.gov
Motivational Interviewing:
  www.motivationalinterview.org
Nasco Nutrition Teaching Aids: www.eNasco.com

Nutrition411: http://nutrition411.com
Nutrition.gov Web site: www.nutrition.gov
Produce for Better Health Nutrition Education:
  www.fruitsandveggiesmorematters.org
US Department of Agriculture. Nutrition Evidence
  Library: www.nel.gov
US Department of Health and Human Services and
  US Department of Agriculture. Dietary Guidelines for
  Americans, 2010: www.dietaryguidelines.gov

LIPID DISORDERS

Academy of Nutrition and Dietetics:
  • Disorders of Lipid Metabolism Evidence-Based
    Nutrition Practice Guidelines:
    www.andevidencelibrary.com/topic.cfm?cat=2659
  • Nutrition Care Manual: www.nutritioncaremanual
    .org (select Diseases/Conditions: Cardiovascular
    Disease: Cerebrovascular Disease, Coronary Artery
    Disease, Disorders of Lipid Metabolism, Heart
    Failure, Hypertension; Metabolic Syndrome)
  • Sports, Cardiovascular, and Wellness Nutrition
    Practice Group: www.scandpg.org

American College of Cardiology: www.acc.org
American Heart Association:
  • Web site: www.americanheart.org
  • My American Heart for Professionals: http://my
    .americanheart.org/portal/professional

Centers for Disease Control and Prevention:
  • Cholesterol: www.cdc.gov/cholesterol
  • Fact Sheets: www.cdc.gov/dhdsp/library/fact_sheets
    .htm
  • Heart Disease: www.cdc.gov/HeartDisease/index.htm

Mediterranean Diet Pyramid: www.oldwayspt.org/med_
    pyramid.html
National Guideline Clearinghouse—Cardiovascular Dis-
    eases: www.guideline.gov/browse/browsemode.aspx
    ?node=4445&type=1
National Heart, Lung, and Blood Institute—Educational
    Materials: www.nhlbi.nih.gov/health/public/web/
    index.htm
National Lipid Associaton: www.lipid.org
Third Report of the Expert Panel on Detection, Evalu-
    ation, and Treatment of High Blood Cholesterol in
    Adults (Adult Treatment Panel III): www.nhlbi.nih
    .gov/guidelines/cholesterol/index.htm

HYPERTENSION

Academy of Nutrition and Dietetics:
- Hypertension Evidence-Based Nutrition Practice
    Guidelines: http://www.andevidencelibrary.com/
    topic.cfm?cat=3260
- Nutrition Care Manual: www.nutritioncaremanual
    .org (Select Diseases/Conditions: Cardiovascular
    Disease: Hypertension)

American Heart Association High Blood Pressure
    Resources for Professionals: www.americanheart.org/
    presenter.jhtml?identifier=2125
American Society of Hypertension: www.ash-us.org
Baylor College of Medicine—Hypertension online: www
    .hypertensiononline.org
Centers for Disease Control and Prevention:
- Fact Sheets: www.cdc.gov/dhdsp/library/fact_sheets
    .htm
- Hypertension: www.cdc.gov/bloodpressure

The National Campaign to Control Hypertension: www
.controlhypertension.org/patient

National Guideline Clearinghouse—Hypertension:
www.guideline.gov/summary/summary.aspx?doc_id
=12817&nbr=6619&ss=6&xl=999

National Heart, Lung, and Blood Institute—National
High Blood Pressure Education Program: www.nhlbi
.nih.gov/about/nhbpep

DIABETES TREATMENT

Academy of Nutrition and Dietetics:
- Diabetes Type 1 and 2 for Adults Evidence-Based
  Nutrition Practice Guidelines:
  www.andevidencelibrary.com/topic.cfm?cat=3253
- Food Nutrient Data for *Choose Your Foods: Exchange
  Lists for Diabetes, 2007* (Exchange Lists by Food
  Group): www.eatright.org/HealthProfessionals/
  content.aspx?id=101&terms=choose+your+foods+
  exchange+list.
- Gestational Diabetes Mellitus (GDM) Evidence-
  Based Nutrition Practice Guidelines:
  http://andevidencelibrary.com/topic.cfm?format_
  tables=0&cat=3731
- Nutrition Care Manual: www.nutritioncaremanual
  .org (Select Diseases/Conditions: Gestational
  Diabetes; Reactive Hypoglycemia [non-diabetic];
  Type 1; Type 2)
- Diabetes Care and Education Practice Group
  (DCE): www.dce.org
- Diabetes Care and Education Group Patient
  Education Handouts: www.dce.org/pub_publications/
  education.asp

American Association of Diabetes Educators (AADE): www.diabeteseducator.org

American Diabetes Association:
- Web site: www.diabetes.org
- American Diabetes Association for Professionals: http://professional.diabetes.org/Default.aspx
- Diabetes and Cardiovascular Disease Toolkit: http://professional.diabetes.org/ResourcesForProfessionals.aspx?typ=17&cid=60425
- Resources for Professionals: http://professional.diabetes.org/ResourcesForProfessionals.aspx?typ=17&cid=60378

Centers for Disease Control and Prevention Diabetes Public Health Resource: www.cdc.gov/diabetes

Diabetes Education Society: www.diabetesedu.org

Diabetes Voice (published quarterly in English, French, Spanish, and Russian): www.diabetesvoice.org

Healthy Diabetes Plate (Idaho Plate Method Study):
- Raidl M, Spain K, Lanting R, Lockard M, Johnson S, Spencer M, et al. The Healthy Diabetes Plate. *Prev Chronic Dis.* 2007. www.cdc.gov/pcd/issues/2007/jan/06_0050.htm
- University of Idaho Extension: What Is the Healthy Diabetes Plate? www.extension.uidaho.edu/diabetesplate/index.html

International Diabetes Center: www.idcpublishing.com

Joslin Diabetes Center Resources for Healthcare Professionals: www.joslin.org/846_4728.asp

Merck's Diabetes Conversation Maps: www.journeyforcontrol.com/journey_for_control/journeyforcontrol/for_educators/conversation_maps

National Diabetes Education Program (NDEP): www.ndep.nih.gov

National Guideline Clearinghouse—Diabetes Mellitus:
   www.guideline.gov/browse/browsemode.aspx?node=
   7546&type=1

National Institute on Aging—Diabetes in Older People:
   www.nia.nih.gov/HealthInformation/Publications/
   diabetes.htm

Potluck Puzzles—Diabetes and Nutrition Education
   Tools: www.potluckpuzzles.com

Present Diabetes: www.presentdiabetes.com

Wellness Proposals Multicultural Diabetes Education
   materials (more than 10 different languages):
   www.wellnessproposals.com/health-care/diabetes
   -handbook-and-resources.htm

DIABETES PREVENTION

Diabetes Prevention Program Lifestyle Materials: http://
   diabetes.niddk.nih.gov/dm/pubs/preventionprogram

National Diabetes Education Program: www.ndep.nih.gov

WEIGHT MANAGEMENT

Academy of Nutrition and Dietetics:
   • Adult Weight Management Evidence-Based Nutrition
     Practice Guidelines: http://www.andevidencelibrary
     .com/topic.cfm?cat=2801
   • Nutrition Care Manual: www.nutritioncaremanual
     .org (Select Diseases/Conditions: Bariatric Surgery;
     Overweight & Obesity; Underweight)
   • Weight Management Practice Group: www.wmdpg
     .org

Body mass index calculators:
   • Centers for Disease Control and Prevention:
     www.cdc.gov/nccdphp/dnpa/bmi

• National Heart, Lung, and Blood Institute: www.nhlbsupport.com/bmi

Centers for Disease Control and Prevention:
  • Overweight and Obesity: www.cdc.gov/obesity/index.html
  • Resources: www.cdc.gov/obesity/resources.html

National Weight Control Registry: www.nwcr.ws
Obesity Society: www.obesity.org

SPANISH RESOURCES

American Association of Diabetes Educators—Practice Spanish for Diabetes Educators: www.diabeteseducators.org/ProfessionalResources/products/view.html?target=40&sub1=BOOKS&sub2=Publications

American Diabetes Association:
  • Información en Español: www.diabetes.org/espanol/default.jsp
  • Reducing Cardiometabolic Risk: Patient Education Toolkit: http://professional.diabetes.org/ResourcesForProfessionals.aspx?cid=60379

Batty PA. *Spanish for the Nutrition Professional*. 2nd ed. Chicago, IL: American Dietetic Association; 2009. www.eatright.org/Shop/Product.aspx?id=5013

National Alliance for Hispanic Health: www.hispanichealth.org

National Diabetes Education Program (NDEP) Publications in Spanish: http://ndep.nih.gov/publications/Publicaciones.aspx

Texas Department of State Health Services—Free diabetes education materials for professionals and patients: www.dshs.state.tx.us/diabetes/patient.shtm

Appendix D

Patient Resources

GENERAL NUTRITION AND HEALTH RESOURCES

Academy of Nutrition and Dietetics
- Consumer Resources: www.eatright.org/Public
- Nutrition Care Manual: www.nutritioncaremanual.org
- Nutrition Fact Sheets: www.eatright.org/Public/content.aspx?id=206

Harvard School of Public Health—The Nutrition Source: www.hsph.harvard.edu/nutritionsource

Health and Nutrition Information for Pregnant and Breastfeeding Women: www.ChooseMyPlate.gov/pregnancy-breastfeeding.html

Super Kids Nutrition: www.superkidsnutrition.com

US Department of Health and Human Services and US Department of Agriculture (USDA)—Dietary Guidelines for Americans, 2010: www.dietaryguidelines.gov

USDA MyPlate: www.ChooseMyPlate.gov

Washington State Dairy Council: www.eatsmart.org

RECIPES AND GROCERY SHOPPING RESOURCES

American Diabetes Association's MyFoodAdvisor: http://tracker.diabetes.org

American Heart Association's Delicious Decisions: www.americanheart.org/deliciousdecisions/jsp/home/home.jsp?_requestid=9229544

Centers for Disease Control and Prevention—Fruits and
Veggies Matter: www.fruitsandveggiesmatter.gov
Diabetes Care and Education Practice Group Recipes:
www.dce.org/resources/recipes/archive
Eating Well Magazine: www.eatingwell.com
National Diabetes Education Program Recipe Booklet:
www.ndep.nih.gov/media/MQC_recipebook_english
.pdf

RESTAURANT NUTRITION INFORMATION

Healthy Dining Finder: www.healthydiningfinder.com
(locates specific restaurants and their healthy options
according to nutrition criteria)
Burger King: www.bk.com/en/us/menu-nutrition/full
-menu.html
McDonald's: www.mcdonalds.com/usa/eat/nutrition_
info.html
Starbucks: www.starbucks.com/menu/nutrition
Subway: www.subway.com/nutrition/nutritionlist.aspx
Wendy's: www.wendys.com/food/Menu.jsp

NUTRITION INFORMATION FOR FOODS
FROM ALL SOURCES

Calorie King: www.calorieking.com (allows food searches
of all types, single ingredients or restaurants foods)
LiveStrong.com Calorie Tracker Application:
www.livestrong.com/thedailyplate/iphone-calorie
-tracker

HEALTHY LIFESTYLE TOOLS

My Food Diary: www.myfooddiary.com
SparkPeople: www.sparkpeople.com

DIETARY SUPPLEMENT INFORMATION

Office of Dietary Supplements: http://ods.od.nih.gov

SPANISH RESOURCES

Academy of Nutrition and Dietetics:
- Información de la nutrición en español: www.eatright.org/espanol
- Seleccione Sus Alimentos: Listas de Intercambios para la Diabetes (Choose Your Foods: Exchange Lists for Diabetes in Spanish): www.eatright.org/Shop/Product.aspx?id=4985

American Heart Association:
- Patient Education Materials: http://es.heart.org/dheart/HEARTORG/Conditions/Answers-by-Heart-Fact-Sheets-Multi-language-Information_UCM_314158_Article.jsp

National Diabetes Education Program (NDEP) Recipe Booklet: http://ndep.nih.gov/media/MQC_recipebook_spanish.pdf

National Diabetes Information Clearinghouse: http://diabetes.niddk.nih.gov/spanish/index.asp

Texas Department of State Health Services—Free diabetes education materials for patients and professionals: www.dshs.state.tx.us/diabetes/patient.shtm

LIPID DISORDERS

Academy of Nutrition and Dietetics Nutrition Care Manual: www.nutritioncaremanual.org

American College of Cardiology patient Web site: www.cardiosmart.org

American Heart Association:
- Web site: www.heart.org
- The Bad Fats Brothers: www.heart.org/
  HEARTORG/GettingHealthy/FatsAndOils/
  MeettheFats/The-Bad-Fats-Brothers_UCM_305102
  _Article.jsp
- The Better Fats Sisters: www.heart.org/
  HEARTORG/GettingHealthy/FatsAndOils/
  MeettheFats/The-Better-Fats-Sisters_UCM_305103
  _Article.jsp
- Cholesterol: www.heart.org/HEARTORG/
  GettingHealthy/FatsAndOils/Fats101/
  Cholesterol-Q-A_UCM_304898_Article.jsp
- Consumer and Patient Education Materials:
  www.heart.org/HEARTORG/General/Consumer
  -and-Patient-Education-Materials_UCM_314813
  _Article.jsp
- Heart Hub for Patients: www.hearthub.org
- My Fats Translator: www.myfatstranslator.com
- Tips for Eating Out: www.heart.org/HEARTORG/
  GettingHealthy/NutritionCenter/DiningOut/Dining
  -Out_UCM_304183_SubHomePage.jsp

HYPERTENSION

Academy of Nutrition and Dietetics Nutrition Care
  Manual: www.nutritioncaremanual.org
American Heart Association:
- Heart Hub High Blood Pressure: www.hearthub.org/
  hc-high-blood-pressure.htm
- High Blood Pressure: Every Step Counts:
  www.heart.org/HEARTORG/Conditions/
  HighBloodPressure/High-Blood-Pressure_UCM_
  002020_SubHomePage.jsp

• High Blood Pressure Tools and Resources:
www.heart.org/HEARTORG/Conditions/HighBlood
Pressure/HighBloodPressureToolsResources/High
-Blood-Pressure-Tools-Resources_UCM_002055
_Article.jsp

The DASH Diet Eating Plan (about the diet, recipes and
tips): www.dashdiet.org

DIABETES TREATMENT

Academy of Nutrition and Dietetics:
• Choose Your Foods: Exchange Lists for Diabetes:
www.eatright.org/Shop/Product.aspx?id=4962
• Choose Your Foods: Plan Your Meals.
www.eatright.org/Shop/Product.aspx?id=6442462993
• Count Your Carbs: Getting Started: www.eatright.org/
Shop/Product.aspx?id=6442451915&CatID=252
• Eating Healthy with Diabetes Easy Reading Guide:
www.eatright.org/Shop/Product.aspx?id=4993
• Match Your Insulin to Your Carbs (flexible
insulin plan). www.eatright.org/shop/product.aspx
?id=6442466923
• Nutrition Care Manual: www.nutritioncaremanual
.org

American Diabetes Association: www.diabetes.org
American Heart Association's Heart Hub Diabetes:
www.hearthub.org/hc-diabetes.htm
Centers for Disease Control and Prevention—Diabetes
& Me: www.cdc.gov/diabetes/consumer/index.htm
Diabetes Online Community: http://Tudiabetes.com
Idaho Plate Method: www.platemethod.com
International Diabetes Center: www.idcpublishing.com
Joslin Diabetes Center: www.joslin.org

Learning about Diabetes: www.learningaboutdiabetes.org

National Diabetes Information Clearinghouse:
   http://diabetes.niddk.nih.gov

DIABETES PREVENTION

American Diabetes Association—Prevention:
   www.diabetes.org/diabetes-basics/prevention

Centers for Disease Control and Prevention:
   • Diabetes & Me: www.cdc.gov/diabetes/consumer/
     index.htm
   • Prevent Diabetes: www.cdc.gov/diabetes/consumer/
     prevent.htm

National Diabetes Education Program—More than 50
   ways to Prevent Diabetes: www.ndep.nih.gov/media/
   50Ways_tips.pdf

WEIGHT MANAGEMENT

Academy of Nutrition and Dietetics:
   • Choose Your Foods: Exchange Lists for Weight
     Management: www.eatright.org/Shop/Product.aspx?
     id=6442462970
   • Nutrition Care Manual: www.nutritioncaremanual
     .org

American Heart Association Patient Information Sheets:
   www.heart.org/HEARTORG/Conditions/Answers
   -by-Heart-Fact-Sheets_UCM_300330_Article.jsp

Calories-Count: www.caloriescount.com

Calorie King: www.calorieking.com

Change One from Reader's Digest: www.changeone.com

eDiets: www.ediets.com

FitDay: www.fitday.com

Men's Health Personal Trainer: www.mhpersonaltrainer
　　.com/uof/mhpersonaltrainer/50373/index.html
My Diet (MiDieta): www.midieta.com
My Food Diary: www.myfooddiary.com
Nutrition.gov Weight Management: www.nutrition.gov/
　　nal_display/index.php?info_center=11&tax_level=1
　　&tax_subject=390
Portion Distortion: http://hp2010.nhlbihin.net/portion/
Spark People: www.sparkpeople.com
Volumetrics: www.volumetricseatingplan.com/
WebMD Weight Loss Clinic: www.weightloss.webmd
　　.com
Weight Control Information Network: http://win.niddk
　　.nih.gov/index.htm
Weight Watchers: www.weightwatchers.com

References

1. Academy of Nutrition and Dietetics. Evidence Analysis Library. http://www.andevidencelibrary.com. Accessed March 5, 2012.

2. Academy of Nutrition and Dietetics. *International Dietetics & Nutrition Terminology (IDNT) Reference Manual. Standardized Language for the Nutrition Care Process.* 4th ed. Chicago, IL: Academy of Nutrition and Dietetics; 2013.

3. American Dietetic Association Quality Management Committee. American Dietetic Association revised 2008 standards of practice for registered dietitians in nutrition care; standards of professional performance for registered dietitians; standards of practice for dietetic technicians, registered, in nutrition care; and standards of professional performance for dietetic technicians, registered. *J Am Diet Assoc.* 2008;108:1538–1542.

4. Nutrition Care Process SNAPshots. http://www.eatright.org/HealthProfessionals/content.aspx?id=5902&terms=Nutrition+Care+Process+SNAPshots. Accessed May 20, 2010.

5. Academy of Nutrition and Dietetics. Disorders of Lipid Metabolism Evidence-Based Nutrition Practice Guidelines. http://www.andevidencelibrary.com/topic.cfm?cat=2659. 2011. Accessed March 5, 2012.

6. Academy of Nutrition and Dietetics. Hypertension Evidence-Based Nutrition Practice Guidelines. 2008. http://www.andevidencelibrary.com/topic.cfm?cat=3260. Accessed March 5, 2012.

7. Academy of Nutrition and Dietetics. Diabetes Type 1 and 2 for Adults Evidence-Based Nutrition Practice Guidelines. 2008. http://www.andevidencelibrary.com/topic.cfm?cat=3253. Accessed March 5, 2012.

8. Franz MJ, Powers MA, Leontos C, Holzmeister LA, Kulkarni K, Monk A, Wedel N, Gradwell E. The evidence for medical nutrition therapy for type 1 and type 2 diabetes in adults. *J Am Diet Assoc.* 2010;110:1852–1859.

9. Academy of Nutrition and Dietetics. Gestational Diabetes Mellitus (GDM) Evidence-Based Nutrition Practice Guidelines. http://andevidencelibrary.com/topic.cfm?format_tables=0&cat=3731. 2008. Accessed March 5, 2012.

10. Academy of Nutrition and Dietetics. Adult Weight Management Evidence-Based Nutrition Practice Guidelines. 2006. http://www.andevidencelibrary.com/topic.cfm?cat=2801. Accessed March 5, 2012.

11. Expert Panel on Detection, Evaluation, and Treatment of High Blood Cholesterol in Adults. Executive summary of the third report of the National Cholesterol Education Program (NCEP) Expert Panel on Detection, Evaluation, and Treatment of High Blood Cholesterol in Adults (Adult Treatment Panel III). *JAMA.* 2001;285:2486–2497; update *Circulation.* 2004;110:227–239.

12. Grundy SM, Cleeman JI, Daniels SR, Donato KA, Eckel RH, Franklin BA, Gordon DJ, Krauss RM, Savage PH, Smith SC, Spertus JA, Costa F. Diagnosis and management of the metabolic syndrome. An American Heart Association/National Heart, Lung, and Blood Institute Scientific Statement. *Circulation.* 2005;112:2735–2752.

13. Appel LJ, Brands MW, Daniels SR, Karanja N, Elmer PJ, Sacks FM. Dietary approaches to prevent and treat hypertension. A scientific statement from the American Heart Association. *Hypertension.* 2006;47:296–308.

14. The Seventh Report of the Joint National Committee on Prevention, Detection, Evaluation and Treatment of High Blood Pressure: The JNC 7 Report. *JAMA.* 2003;289:2560–2572.

15. American Diabetes Association. Standards of medical care in diabetes—2012. *Diabetes Care.* 2012;35(suppl 1):S11–S63.

16. Garber AJ, Handelsman Y, Einhorn D, Bergman DA, Bloomgarden ZT, Fonseca V, Garvey WT, Gavin JR 3rd, Grunberg G, Horton ES, Jellinger PS, Jones KL, Lebovitz H, Levy P, McGuire DK, Moghissi ES, Nesto RW. Diagnosis and management of prediabetes in the continuum of hyperglycemia: when do the risks of diabetes begin? A consensus statement from the American College of Endocrinology and the American Association of Clinical Endocrinologists. *Endocr Pract.* 2008;7:933-946.

17. National Heart, Lung, and Blood Institute. *Clinical Guidelines on the Identification, Evaluation and Treatment of Overweight and Obesity in Adults.* Bethesda, MD: National Institutes of Health; 1998.

18. US Department of Health and Human Services. 2008 Physical Activity Guidelines for Americans. http://www.health.gov/paguidelines. Accessed March 5, 2012.

19. American College of Sports Medicine. Appropriate physical activity intervention strategies for weight loss and prevention of weight regain for adults. *Med Sci Sports Exerc.* 2009;41:459–471.

20. Van Horn L, McCoin M, Kris-Etherton PM, Burke F, Carson JS, Champagne CM, Karmally W, Sikand G. The evidence for dietary prevention and treatment of cardiovascular disease. *J Am Diet Assoc.* 2008;108:287–331.

21. Chobanian AV, Bakris GL, Black HR, Cushman WC, Green LA, Izzo JK Jr, Jones DW, Materson BJ, Oparil S, Wright JT Jr, Roccella EJ; National Heart, Lung, and Blood Institute Joint National Committee on Prevention, Detection, Evaluation, and Treatment of High Blood Pressure; National High Blood Pressure Education Program Coordinating Committee. The Seventh Report of the Joint National Committee on Prevention, Detection, Evaluation and Treatment of High Blood Pressure: The JNC 7 report. *JAMA.* 2003;289:2560–2572.

22. Appel LJ, Champagne CM, Harsha DW, Cooper LS, Obarzanek E, Elmer PJ, Stevens VJ, Vollmer WM, Lin PH, Svetkey LP, Stedman SW, Young DR, for the Writing Groups of the PREMIER Collaborative Research Group. Effects of comprehensive lifestyle modification on blood pressure control: main results of the PREMIER clinical trial. *JAMA.* 2003;289:2083–2093.

23. Academy of Nutrition and Dietetics Evidence Analysis Library. Effectiveness of MNT for hypertension. http://www.andevidence library.com/conclusion.cfm?conclusion_statement_id=251204. Accessed May 20, 2010.

24. Franz MJ, Boucher JL, Green-Pastors J, Powers MA. Evidence-based nutrition practice guidelines for diabetes and scope and standards of practice. *J Am Diet Assoc.* 2008;108:S52–S58.

25. Klein S, Sheard NF, Pi-Sunyer X, Daly A, Wylie-Rosett J, Kulkarni K, Clark NG. Weight management through lifestyle modification for the prevention and management of type 2 diabetes: rationale and strategies. *Diabetes Care.* 2004;27:2067–2073.

26. Knowler WC, Barrett-Connor E, Fowler SE, Hamman RF, Lachin JM, Walker EA, Nathan DM. Reduction in the incidence of type 2 diabetes with lifestyle intervention or metformin. *N Engl J Med.* 2002;346:393–403.

27. Diabetes Prevention Program Research Group. 10-year follow-up of diabetes incidence and weight loss in the Diabetes Prevention Program Outcome Study. *Lancet.* 2009;374:1677–1686.

28. Lindström J, Ilanne-Parikka P, Peltonen M, Aunola S, Eriksson JG, Hämäläinen H, Härkönen P, Keinänen-Kiukaanniemi S, Laakso M, Louheranta A, Mannelin M, Paturi M, Sundvall J, Valle TT, Uusitupa M, Tuomilehto J; Finnish Diabetes Prevention Study Group. Sustained reduction in the incidence of type 2 diabetes by lifestyle intervention: follow-up of the Finnish Diabetes Prevention Study. *Lancet.* 2006;368:1673–1679.

29. Seagle HM, Strain GW, Makris A, Reeves RS. Position of the American Dietetic Association: weight management. *J Am Diet Assoc.* 2009;109:330–346.

30. Franz MJ, VanWormer JJ, Crain L, Boucher JL, Histon T, Caplan W, Bowman JD, Pronk NP. Weight-loss outcomes: a systematic review and meta-analysis of weight-loss clinical trials with a minimum 1-year follow-up. *J Am Diet Assoc.* 2007;107:1755–1767.

31. Academy of Nutrition and Dietetics Evidence Analysis Library. Effectiveness of MNT for Obesity. http://www.andevidence library.com/topic.cfm?cat=4171. Accessed March 5, 2012.

32. Klein S, Burke LE, Gray GA, Glair S, Allison DB, Pi-Sunyer X, Hong Y, Eckel RH. Clinical implications of obesity with specific focus on cardiovascular disease. A statement for professionals from the American Heart Association Council on Nutrition, Physical Activity, and Metabolism. *Circulation.* 2004;110:2952–2967.

33. Third Report of the Expert Panel on Detection, Evaluation, and Treatment of High Blood Cholesterol in Adults (Adult Panel III). Bethesda, MD: National Institutes of Health, National Heart, Lung, and Blood Institute; 2001. NIH publication 01-3670.

34. Myers GL, Rifai N, Tracy RP, Roberts WL, Alexander RW, Biasucci LM, Catravas JD, Cole TG, Cooper GR, Khan BV, Kimberly MM, Stein EA, Taubert KA, Warnick R, Waymack PP. CDC/AHA Workshop on markers of inflammation and cardiovascular disease: application to clinical and public health practice: report from the Laboratory Science Discussion Group. *Circulation.* 2004;110:e545–e549.

35. Alberti KGMM, Eckel RH, Grundy SM, Zimmet PZ, Cleeman JI, Donato KA, Fruchart JC, James PT, Loria CM, Smith Jr, SC. Harmonizing the metabolic syndrome. A Joint Interim Statement of the International Diabetes Federation Task Force on Epidemiology and Prevention; National Heart, Lung and Blood Institute;

American Heart Association; World Health Federation; International Atherosclerosis Society; and International Association for the Study of Obesity. *Circulation.* 2009;120:1640–1645.

36. The Seventh Report of the Joint National Committee on Prevention, Detection, Evaluation and Treatment of High Blood Pressure: The JNC 7 Report. Bethesda, MD: National Institutes of Heart, Lung, and Blood Institute; 2003. NIH publication 03-5231.

37. American Dietetic Association. *Adult Weight Management Toolkit.* Chicago, IL: American Dietetic Association; 2007.

38. Haskell WL, Lee I-M, Pate RR, Powell KE, Blair SN, Franklin BA, Macera CA, Heath GW, Thompson PD, Bauman A. Physical activity and public health. Updated recommendations for adults from the American College of Sports Medicine and the American Heart Association. *Circulation.* 2007;116:1081–1093.

39. Kaufman FR, ed. *Medical Management of Type 1 Diabetes.* 5th ed. Alexandria, VA: American Diabetes Association; 2008.

40. Spahn JM, Reeves RS, Keim KS, Laquatra I, Kellogg M, Jortberg B, Clark NA. State of the evidence regarding behavior change theories and strategies in nutrition counseling to facilitate health and food behavior change. *J Am Diet Assoc.* 2010;110:879–891.

41. Artinian NT, Fletcher GF, Mozaffarian D, Kris-Etherton P, Van Horn L, Lichtenstein AH, Kumanyika S, Kraus WE, Fleg JL, Redeker NS, Meininger JC, Banks J, Stuart-Shor EM, Fletcher BJ, Miller TD, Hughes S, Braun LT, Kopin LA, Berra K, Hayman LL, Ewing LJ, Ades PA, Durstine JL, Houston-Miller N, Burke LE; on behalf of the American Heart Association Prevention Committee of the Council on Cardiovascular Nursing. Interventions to promote physical activity and dietary lifestyle changes for cardiovascular risk factor reduction in adults. A Scientific Statement from the American Heart Association. *Circulation.* 2010;122:406–441.

42. VanWormer JJ, Boucher JL. The 5 A's: behavior change counseling in the context of brief clinical encounters. *On the Cutting Edge: Diabetes Care and Education.* 2003;24(4):24–26.

43. VanWormer JJ, Boucher JL. Motivational interviewing and diabetes education: fostering commitment to change. *On the Cutting Edge: Diabetes Care and Education.* 2003;24(4):14–16.

44. VanWormer JJ, Boucher JL. Motivational interviewing and diet modification: a review of the evidence. *Diabetes Educator.* 2004;30:404–419.

45. Prochaska JO, Velicer WF. The transtheoretical model of health behavior changes. *Am J Health Promotion.* 1997;12:38–48.

46. Gehling E. Changing us or changing them? *Newsflash (*newsletter of the Diabetes Care and Education Practice Group of the American Dietetic Association). 1999;20:31–33.

47. Klein S, Burke LE, Gray GA, Glair S, Allison DB, Pi-Sunyer X, Hong Y, Eckel RH. Clinical implications of obesity with specific focus on cardiovascular disease. A statement for professionals from the American Heart Association Council on Nutrition, Physical Activity, and Metabolism. *Circulation.* 2004;110:2952–2967.

48. Yu-Poth S, Zhao G, Etherton T, Naglak M, Jonnalagadda S, Kris-Etherton PM. Effects of the National Cholesterol Education Program's Step I and Step II dietary intervention programs on cardiovascular disease risk factors: a meta-analysis. *Am J Clin Nutr.* 1999;69:632–646 .

49. Writing Group of the Nutrition Care Process/Standardized Language Committee. Nutrition Care Process Part II: Using the International Dietetics and Nutrition Terminology to document the Nutrition Care Process. *J Am Diet Assoc.* 2008;108:1287–1293.

50. Frankenfield D, Roth-Yousey L, Compher C. Comparison of predictive equations for resting metabolic rate in healthy non-obese and obese adults: a systematic review. *J Am Diet Assoc.* 2005;105:775–778.

51. International Diabetes Center. *Guide to Starting and Adjusting Insulin for Type 2 Diabetes.* Minneapolis, MN: International Diabetes Center at Park Nicollet; 2006.

Index

Page number followed by *t* indicates table.